What People Are Saying At

"Kristy is an inspiration to us all. I've had the opportunity to work closely with her throughout her heart journey. Her servant leadership, dedication, and passion were clearly evident from our first meeting. Fast forward through Kristy's additional heart challenges, and she has used her story to move others to take action. Kristy is an overcomer, and a passionate volunteer leader for a lifesaving mission. Courageously sharing her personal story will show survivors that they are not alone and that they, too, can overcome and inspire others. Thank you, Kristy!"

— Kevin Harker
Executive Vice President, Midwest Region
American Heart Association

"Project Beautiful – Inside and Out was honored to have Kristy preview her book, *Change of Heart*, as part of our 'Building Confidence, Inspiring Hope' Speaker Series. It was an amazing evening working through Kristy's Wellness Widget — including introspection exercises, a group meditation, plenty of laughs, and even a few tears. Her journey, positive attitude, and unstoppable energy are truly inspiring!"

— Doris Gilles
Executive Director of Project Beautiful – Inside and Out

"I have so much admiration for the way Kristy is using the power of her story to help others. By authentically sharing her remarkable recovery experience, she's truly helping to change the concept of wellness."

— Kristi Piehl
Founder & CEO: Media Minefield & Host of Flip Your Script

"Kristy has taught me much about how to approach life's challenges with bravery and positivity. Her optimism is infectious and her resilience in overcoming setbacks provides a successful formula for those wanting to live a more fearless and fulfilled life."

— Allison Robinson
Founder and CEO of The Mom Project

"How can you not think about your own health when watching Kristy's journey? After stepping away from the C-suite, I knew it was time to get my physical self together. Kristy's journey encouraged me to work out more, eat better, and most importantly... just find my joy.

If everybody could appreciate life like Kristy, we would have a more joyful society. When you meet her and hear her story, you're mesmerized about how positive she was and is about every step of her journey. You can't help but walk away saying 'I need to be more like Kristy.'"

— Teresa Carroll
Board Director, Strategic Advisor, Former President

"To say Kristy is a true inspiration hardly does her justice. Kristy's drive, positive energy, and self-motivation would be spectacular without her amazing back story. What is even more impressive is the impact she has had on literally hundreds of people all over the world who have benefited from experiencing her contagious uplifting spirit. Truly, the power of the universe personified!"

— Bruce Morton
Global Workforce Strategist and Author

"Kristy is an exemplar of resilience, strength, and grit. She has struggled with heart disease for more than 20 years, culminating in a recent heart transplant. Her passion to raise awareness for heart disease is only rivaled by her optimism that powered her through a swift transplant recovery. Kristy's story is inspiring, and she has plenty of hard-won wisdom to share."

— Greg Brown, CFP®
Founder, Pathway Financial Planning, LLC

"I can truly say that Kristy exudes one of the most positive outlooks I have ever seen. The last few years of her life would have proved a challenge for most, but they have only deepened her spirit, zest for life, and passion for living. I am blessed to have known her for over thirty years, and she continues to inspire me to this day!"

— MJ LaDuke
Certified Yoga Instructor

"She had an enormously large heart, but it functioned poorly. She lived a vigorous and accomplished life knowing full well that it would be severely compromised without a new heart. Kristy Sidlar writes with clarity and candor about her recovery following a heart transplant. Her views on how to successfully navigate the journey from ill-health to wellness has much to teach all of us."

— Creig Hoyt, MD, MA
Department of Ophthalmology
University of California, San Francisco

"Kristy epitomizes determination, strength, and grit. She persevered with her heart disease diagnosis as a fit and vibrant young woman and used it as her driving force to bring awareness to others, especially women. Since receiving her new heart and new lease on life, she is stronger, fitter, and more determined than ever to live her best, healthiest life. She is an inspiration to all and embodies the true meaning of fitness."

— Nancy Kilcullen, MS, CPT
Exercise Physiologist and Personal Trainer

"It is a blessing that Kristy is sharing with us the insight she has gained from a second chance with her new heart! As someone who has struggled with heart disease myself, it is so important to hear Kristy's message of HOPE. Kristy's wellness dimensions emphasize the need to have a multi-pronged approach to healing."

— Herman Williams, MD, MBA, MPH
Author and Chief Physician Executive
Hardenbergh Group

"Kristy is intellectual, insightful, and pragmatic. This was clearly reflected by how she approached her recovery from more of an information-rich angle. I loved how she kept her circle of people updated constantly, to include her wins and her struggles, on a daily basis after her surgery. It is so exciting to see her live life like nothing ever happened. Her book and her stories can give hope to many. I can't wait to follow her striking victories in the great war of life."

— Manish Senta, PhD, PMP
Managing Director of TEKWISSEN

"Kristy Sidlar is a kind, honest, and engaging young woman who dealt with a life-threatening health condition with dignity and a positive attitude. Since the transplant, Kristy is still that same person but with renewed energy and purpose. She has created a practical application of wellness that I think any psychotherapist would find helpful working with their clients."

— Richard Paritzky
Licensed Clinical Psychologist

"Seeing the world through the eyes of Kristy, a heart transplant survivor, was deeply inspiring. She has a fighting spirit balanced with a pragmatic 'one day at a time' approach. I also enjoy her absolute transparency and transformative style.

Her acceptance of her reality and the bravery she exhibits put all other challenges in one's life into perspective."

— Ralph Gilles
Friend and Chief Design Officer of Stellantis

"When I work with my clients, in addition to nutrition, sleep, exercise, etc., I encourage an understanding of the importance of mindset. Kristy is such a strong example of valuing this view. Her clean living and positive mindset moved her through to a full and joyful recovery. I am so excited she is sharing her incredible journey with the world!"

— Dr. Debbie Moffatt, ND

"Kristy has done remarkably well after her heart transplant. She recovered at a rate faster than many patients and is thriving with her new heart. Part of her success after transplant must be due to her mindset. She came into this major life crisis with a 'can do' attitude and kept fighting. She conquered death with a transplant but did not become complacent thereafter. She has continued to strive for a healthy lifestyle. Her spirit, optimism, and zeal are amazing and must play a positive role in her health."

— Jennifer Cowger, MD, MS, FACC
Kristy's Transplant Doctor

"The way Kristy approaches life is truly nothing short of amazing. A transplant will shift anyone's perspective, but what's really special about Kristy is she lived every day and took care of her health, just as authentic and optimistic before, as she does now after her transplant. A true inspiration, and there is nothing she can't overcome."

— Katy Saltsman
Nutritionist and Personal Trainer

"'Kristy's heart is too big.' I've always thought this about my dear friend, but never did I think that would be her official medical condition when first meeting her in 1987. I have had a front row seat to watch Kristy fight from diagnosis to transplant. Her grit and determination to regain her health is inspiring. This book will inspire you to examine your life's priorities and what matters most. My dear friend and her warrior heart's story will inspire you to be a better version of yourself as you laugh and cry and many other emotions in between. The planet is a much better place with Kristy and her giant (now normal sized) heart. Some stories are just made to be shared, and Kristy's is absolutely one of those stories."

— Andrea Schmitz
Licensed Marriage and Family Therapist, and College Roommate

"Kristy is an absolute rock star! I am awed and honored to help her present this book to the world, because her powerful testimony will inspire people everywhere. Since our first book coaching session, to the completion and publication of this book, Kristy has done what so many people talk about, but never do: commit their stories to the pages of a book. This courageous act leaves a legacy, and provides a teaching tool to serve as a way-shower. So let Kristy inspire you to preserve your story in a book, because you may improve — or even save — a life by sharing what you know. Her personality sparkles through her storytelling, and she handles grim material in a way that makes you smile, laugh, cry, and keep turning the pages. I'm proud to call Kristy a friend, and I hope you enjoy reading this book as much as I enjoyed helping her create it! Congratulations, Kristy!"

— Elizabeth Ann Atkins
America's Book Coach
CEO, Two Sisters Writing & Publishing

CHANGE OF HEART

My Journey of Transplantation, Revelation & Transformation

KRISTY SIDLAR

CHANGE OF HEART:
My Journey of Transplantation, Revelation & Transformation
Kristy Sidlar
Copyright © 2022 Kristy Sidlar
All Rights Reserved.

For information about this title or to order other books and/or electronic media, contact the publisher:

Atkins & Greenspan Publishing
TwoSistersWriting.com
18530 Mack Avenue, Suite 166
Grosse Pointe Farms, MI 48236

ISBN 978-1-956879-03-2 (Hardcover)
ISBN 978-1-956879-04-9 (Paperback)
ISBN 978-1-956879-05-6 (eBook)

Printed in the United States of America

All the stories in this work are true.

Cover and Interior Design: Graphic designer Michelle Halliday, Illustrator Jodi Burton, and Van-garde Imagery, Inc.

Photo credit for author photo: Greg Sadler.

All photographs used with permission.

All uncredited photographs courtesy of the Sidlar Family Collection.

This book is dedicated to:

Warren "Chip" Brown
&
Catherine Laurencelle

Chip, my uncle, and Catherine, one of my dearest friends, were both exceptionally active and seemingly very healthy people. Both died of massive heart attacks during the time I wrote this book.

Advocacy for heart health has been my mission for more than 20 years.

Because of these two unexpected and unnecessary deaths, I invite you to please ask your doctor about getting a coronary calcium scan. It is a simple, inexpensive, non-invasive test that identifies and measures blockage (calcium build-up) in your arteries.

Blockage is the most common cause of a heart attack. Please take this simple step, for yourself and your loved ones.

Prologue

I'M THE ETERNAL OPTIMIST. Maybe even a bit Pollyanna. My glass is half full. I look for the silver lining. There's always a bright side. I don't worry, unless there's something to worry about. Maybe my perpetually positive attitude led me to be too trusting or blinded in some situations, but generally speaking, in the game of life, I'm winning... definitely winning! When the universe served up my life or death options... no doubt winning was the side I wanted to be on. And win I did!

Allow me to take you on my journey of narrow escapes, life choices, attitude adjustments, and a second chance at living that, as hard as it is for me to fathom, will be better than my first chance. Yep — that eternal optimism burns bright, and as for Kristy 2.0... this upgrade is going to be so worth the wait.

What you are about to read is based on me living through and coming out the very successful end of a not-so-pleasant, 22-year cardiac experience. But my message is not strictly about my heart disease; it is about why my journey was so successful, why my focus on the core dimensions of wellness made my living with heart disease and beating it possible, why doctors tell the story of Kristy Sidlar and her recovery being like few they have seen.

I believe we have a personal responsibility to our bodies, our loved ones, our healthcare system, and our future. And although I don't purport to have done everything right, I do believe I learned some very valuable lessons along the way that I feel obligated to share. I want others to be able to make a positive impact on their own health and on the people who want to see them live a long, fulfilling life.

Take some or all of what I share with you to heart. Whether you choose one single thing to change, or you voraciously devour all my advice, either choice means progress. And if I can help you or your mom or your best friend or your brother make more revolutions around the sun, then I have done what I set out to do by writing this book.

— Kristy Sidlar

Contents

Chapter 1 – The Beginning

SO PICTURE THIS. YOU'RE in a fitness class. Your instructor is 30 minutes into the session. Energy is high. She goes to grab for her bottle of water — not something she typically does in the middle of a complicated step sequence.

Then *bam!* She passes out.

As the students recall the story, the fainting wasn't really a crumpled thud. It was like the leading lady of a 1950's movie, hand draped across her forehead, gracefully folding toward the floor. Graceful maybe, but definitely out cold.

That instructor was me back in April of 1996. I had taught hundreds of classes, but for some unknown reason on that day, my body was not up for it. Maybe it was revolting against hearing Salt-N-Pepa's *Push It* one too many times!

I got exceptionally lightheaded during the peak intensity of the class. Next thing you know, I woke up to two very handsome EMTs staring down at me. I was a little dazed and confused, but honestly not all that disappointed. I was happy to take in the scenery for a little longer!

And here's a funny side note to this story. As soon as I passed out, one of my students called our Saturday on-call manager, and told her, "Kristy just passed out in front of the class!"

The manager (I'll call her Sylvia to save her any embarrassment when she buys this book for everyone she knows), was an absolute prankster and loved April Fool's jokes. Sylvia had ironically just pulled off a very similar prank for the fitness center's owner two weeks before. She had one of the students call the owner to tell her that Sylvia had passed out in front of a class and that she should come to the gym immediately.

The owner arrived to the sight of Sylvia holding a box of donuts, with a shit-eating grin on her face, and crooning a very proud "April Fools' Day!"

So, when Sylvia got the call about ME on April 15, 1996, she laughed and said, "Yeah, whatever!" She didn't realize that I literally was unconscious on the studio floor, probably with a bump on my head and EMTs on the way.

I honestly don't know if they ever convinced her on that call that they were being serious. I do know, however, that after that incident, Sylvia scaled WAY back on her April Fools' Day pranks.

OK, back to me. The paramedics took my vitals and told me I was fine and that I should go to the ER and get checked out. Their rationale was, "You're probably dehydrated, or maybe you didn't eat enough last night."

They said I could potentially have a concussion and gave me all those standard precautions. But the bottom line was, "Nothing is wrong. You can go home."

I never really thought much of it until these similar episodes, although not fully passing out, continued to happen over the course of the next few months. I finally went to the doctor. The ER staff ran several tests, among them an EKG. Once they removed the leads, I got dressed, and the tech gave the printout to the doctor. The doctor said, "This can't be right. Do another one."

They performed another EKG. I got dressed, the tech gave it to the doctor, the doctor said, "This can't be right. Do another one."

They performed a third EKG. This time, my smart genes kicked in and I asked the tech to please give it to the doctor before I got dressed. Yay me, because he did, in fact, order a fourth one.

The doctor said, "This EKG shows she had a heart attack."

I didn't think that was the case, and he wasn't convinced either, but clearly something was wrong. They were scratching their heads; I was confused and naturally concerned. This moment of mutual perplexity began the next several weeks of trying to figure out what was wrong with me.

I was so physically fit back when all this was happening, that I think I out-performed a half a dozen stress tests. We were trying to recreate what happens to me when I am exercising intensely. But short of being at the highest incline and fastest pace (and almost throwing up from over-exertion), we were not successful in identifying the problem.

Until the fateful day I will call "Season 1, Episode 7."

During my seventh stress test my heart finally decided to read the script and cooperate. My heart rate went into overdrive and all of a sudden, I felt like a scene from *ER* (*Grey's Anatomy* had not come out yet, so I'm going old school and referencing George Clooney and Noah Wyle).

All of a sudden, they threw me onto the crash cart, and what seemed like 20 curiosity-seeking doctors and nurses magically appeared in the doorway.

While the medical professionals came at me with the shock paddles, they decided they would first try an injection of lidocaine. Just as they were about to insert the needle, my body converted back to a normal rhythm, and no treatment was necessary.

Hooray!

I was excited because: 1) I survived; 2) I had my normal, comfortable heart beat back; and 3) we had some kind of an answer. Since I was hooked up to the monitors, we could now make a determination about what was going on with my abnormal heart rhythm.

After further evaluation, they diagnosed me with something called right ventricular outflow tract tachycardia (RVOT). They prescribed a beta blocker and advised me not to exercise as intensely as I had been.

My aerobic instructor days had come to an end. Yep, I called myself an aerobic instructor. Remember, this was 1996. To really burn that era and image into your mind, the day I passed out I was wearing a floral thong leotard and matching lilac-colored spandex shorts. Wow! That was the 90's alright.

I stopped teaching classes, I ramped my running down to walking with a little rollerblading for variety (again...so 1990's), and I was told that as suddenly as my RVOT came on, it may go away over time. They advised me to monitor how I felt, and I would be allowed to increase my exercise intensity if my body could tolerate it. Spoiler alert! Giving that kind of permission to somebody who was exercise crazed... probably not the wisest decision.

Shortly after my initial diagnosis, I moved from North Carolina to the San Francisco Bay Area. I was running. I rollerbladed 50 miles from San Francisco to San Jose. I was completing 100-mile bike rides.

And as if that weren't enough, I figured it was time to train for a triathlon.

One Sunday afternoon, I went for a training ride to the gym, where I planned to swim laps and get in a run. That day just happened to be my 31st birthday — October 31, 1999. I was riding my bike, by myself, cresting a hill, when I went into tachycardia. Knowing that my body usually converted out on its own, I sat on my bike for 15 minutes, waiting for my rapid rhythm to go back to normal.

At this point, I was getting a little lightheaded, so I got off my bike and sat on the side of the road. Another 15 minutes passed. I was getting really lightheaded and I needed to lie down. There I was on the shoulder, with my bike by my side.

Remember this was 1999; it was not common practice to carry a cell phone everywhere. So I was lying on by back, by myself, fading in and out of consciousness, wondering if these were going to be my last moments. Some birthday this was turning out to be. Sounded a little more like a cruel joke.

Fortunately, another cyclist came by about five minutes after I went horizontal, and he called the paramedics. I will never EVER forget, in between my moments of consciousness and absolute discomfort, this stranger with his hand on my arm saying, "Stay with us, Kristy. You can do this. Stay awake. The ambulance is almost here."

His words really did make a difference and I often recall that voice and his genuine concern. They arrived quickly, cut my cycling jersey and sports bra off, and applied the defibrillator pads on me. For some reason — another cruel joke — by this point about a dozen other cyclists and runners had shown up and were hovering around me and my bare chest. Fun times! Honestly, them seeing me shirtless was the least of my concerns. I just wanted my normal heartbeat back.

At this point, one of the paramedics (the cuter of the two cuties), said to me, "OK, we're going to defibrillate you. This is going to hurt."

Side note, think about what you see in the movies — almost every time somebody has the shock paddles administered, they're dead. I was very alive (well maybe not very alive, but certainly not dead). He told me he was going to give me some valium to dull the pain, but it was still going to hurt. And then he said, "OK, Here we go."

I braced myself.

What? That was it?

The sensation was so underwhelming compared to what I was preparing myself for. It felt like somebody had lightly pushed their index finger on my chest. I felt next to nothing.

I think they gave me too much Valium. Well, I KNOW they gave me too much Valium because I immediately said in my drug-induced stupor, "Great. Can I ride my bike home now?"

The EMT gave me a very stern look, shook his head, and said, "We just recorded your heart rate at 280 beats per minute. You are going straight to the hospital."

They ran a few tests and declared that, yes, this was the result of the RVOT I was diagnosed with a couple years earlier. Although it was hard to treat just a few short years earlier, the procedure to reverse my funky rhythm was very commonplace now. They released me from the hospital the next morning and told me to make an appointment to get the diseased portion of my ventricle ablated, which is basically cauterizing my abnormal tissue and destroying it, so it can't go haywire and shoot my heartrate up.

"Don't exercise for the rest of the day," the docs said.

I listened to the doctors like a good patient. I did not exercise the rest of the day, but they didn't say I couldn't exercise THE NEXT

DAY, so I went to the gym, got on the treadmill, and started running. I got lightheaded and felt like I was going to pass out. Fortunately, I was able to hit stop on the treadmill panel before that happened. I was promptly taken to the hospital.

I will never forget that night in the ER. They came at me again with the lidocaine to try to slow down my rhythm. This experience was very different from my first one back in 1996. They obviously gave me too much.

"I'm going to die!" I screamed from the ER. "I'm going to die! I'm going to die!"

The lidocaine dosage made everything go black, but I was still conscious. My tongue swelled. I was exceptionally uncomfortable, not to mention scared.

I didn't realize that I was on my way to crushing the ER doctor's fingers until he finally said, "Kristy you have to let go of my hand!"

They were able to convert me out with the injection. At this point, the doctor said, "We are moving you to a room, and you are on hospital arrest until you get this taken care of!"

I assumed I would be there for a couple of days while they performed some tests and the ablation procedure. Ten days (and many tests later) I was diagnosed with a very rare condition called Arrhythmogenic Right Ventricular Cardiomyopathy (ARVC). I quickly learned how incredibly fortunate I was to get this diagnosis when I did. Many people with ARVC experience only one symptom — sudden death.

ARVC essentially makes my healthy right ventricle turn into fatty, fibrous tissue that ultimately will turn into something that looks like a porous sponge. And along the way, my ventricle and eventually my entire heart will continue to enlarge because of how inefficient its pumping ability will be. RVOT was a safe diagnosis based on what my doctors knew back in 1996, but it was definitely a misdiagnosis.

ARVC is a progressive disease. And to my absolute disenchantment, I was told ARVC progresses through exercise. This was one of the worst things they could have told somebody who loves to exercise more than just about anything else in life. Still, I was able to accept the diagnosis; it was the hand I was dealt, and I would make the most of it.

I was fine when they told me that they were going to surgically insert an implantable cardioverter defibrillator (ICD); I was OK with having to take medication for the rest of my life. But when the cardiologist said, "You have to stop training," that's when I lost it. The ugly tears started flowing. Being told I'd have to eliminate something that was so core to my being was one of the hardest things I had ever had to hear.

I got over it pretty quickly. As you will find through many other chapters of this book, I'm a very fast processor. I looked at the bright side and said to myself (and to my mom and the doctors who were in my hospital room with me) something to the effect of:

"Maybe I can't do a triathlon, maybe I can't run any more, but I can walk, I'm alive, and now I can help other people through my experiences."

I wanted to do this in a way that might get people to take action about their own health that they may not have otherwise done without some external motivation.

I pulled up my big girl pants, had my defibrillator implanted, recovered in the hospital for a few days, then went home to live what would become my new normal.

Chapter 2 – The Adjustment

ON NOVEMBER 12, 1999, I left the Kaiser Medical Center in San Jose, California, and headed toward my humble little rented house in Mill Valley. I don't remember much about the drive home, but like many things in my life, I associate poignant moments with music. Burned into my memory are the last two songs that were played on the radio, me in the passenger seat approaching the hill to my house–*Meet Virginia* by Train and *Little Black Backpack* by Stroke 9. Both songs are from Bay Area bands, both on my top 20 playlist of all-time favorite songs.

Confession time–I have dreamed about meeting the lead singer of Train, Pat Monahan, many times since that day. In my dream, I tug on his heart strings, telling him how his voice led the trailer for my "new beginnings" moment, how *Meet Virginia* was my "walk-up music" to my new life. Then he asks me to sing with him in the café where I picture us meeting.

Of course, this has never happened, but Mr. Monahan, if you are reading this book, know that I continue to look for you every time I am in the Bay Area, and someday I plan to make this fantasy a reality. In my dream, you don't cringe at my singing. In reality, it's OK if you do.

I was weak, my already thin frame probably eight pounds lighter than when I entered the hospital. I was tired, and I felt out of sorts not working 12 hours a day. Being unable to jump out of bed and throw my running shoes on was so foreign to me. Of course, my body hardly felt like working myself into a sweat, but I craved it. I couldn't do it if I wanted to, and that was crushing. I was, however, ready to face whatever this new chapter of my life was going to look like.

My recovery included not being able to lift my left arm higher than shoulder-height for six weeks. This was precautionary, so I didn't dislodge the newly implanted leads that connected my defibrillator into my heart. I wore a sling. I slept restlessly. I couldn't shower for a week; I could only take a bath. I had this new bulge in my chest and an unsightly scar—both of which I embraced because I knew they meant I had a new permanent lifesaver living inside my chest. I even named my ICD Mario after one of my paramedics!

By day two, I was able to start taking short walks. They included some slight hills. It was a little defeating, knowing that I wasn't running, but I was moving. I was alive. I had more energy, and I knew I was ready to face this next phase of life.

A couple weeks after my surgery, I visited my medical team. In exchange for them removing the 12 staples from where my defibrillator was implanted, I presented them with dozens of heart-shaped cookies decorated with little scars and words of gratitude. How do you thank someone properly for changing the trajectory of your life? Cookies seemed like the best I could do at the moment.

I went back to work. I felt so ready! Until I walked across the office and pulled open a file cabinet drawer for the first time. Again, defeated. I felt like I needed to go home and get back to bed. It's amazing how much energy healing takes out of you. Recovery definitely took a little bit longer than I had planned, but my energy level continued to improve and I was back to normal soon enough — so normal that I figured, why not start running again?

Running... the one thing the doctors told me I should not do any longer if I didn't want my disease to progress any more significantly. Three weeks and I was already forgetting that sage wisdom I had vowed to heed when I was in the hospital. I said I would walk. I said I would do yoga. I said I could handle not going back to my old ways of intense exercise.

My mind just wanted to do more than my body was up to. So one day, I drove into San Francisco. I took a run through Crissy Field along the San Francisco Bay. I was halfway into my three-mile route.

Next thing I knew, I was looking up at the sky, flat on my back on the running path, with several strangers staring down at me. Fortunately, two of them were doctors.

"Do you have a heart condition?" they asked.

I wondered how they knew.

"Do you have a defibrillator?" they asked.

I wondered how they knew.

"We saw your body jolt and assumed you had been shocked," they said.

Yup! That's what happened, alright. And there I was, a mile-and-a-half from my car. I picked myself up, massaged the tender spot on the back of my head where I fell, and *walked* my ass back to the parking lot.

I probably started walking a little more and running a little less after that incident. Maybe. I like to tell myself I listened to my doctors. But if I'm honest and I dig back into the memory bank, every time I felt like things were more normal, I probably found a way to convince myself that it was OK to start running again.

Some people have a hard time quitting smoking. Some can't give up fast food. I couldn't give up running. It sucked so bad to be the person who loved to exercise, but was being told she couldn't. I will admit to having a brief woe-is-me moment.

I asked the Universe, *Why can't you give this stupid disease to someone who would gladly opt for perpetual time in front of the TV?*

Here's why this pull to continue to exercise was a problem. My ARVC diagnosis was very rare and still relatively new in 2000, and a lot of questions remained around the impact of exercise. Most medical journals said that intense exercise — and some even said *any* exercise — progressed the disease to the point that it was recommended that no ARVC patient exercise at all. And then there was the study that said croquet was OK, but not table tennis; it was too intense.

Oh boy. Are you kidding me? Croquet? Who plays croquet? That seemed a little extreme.

As I think back, I'm sure I just tried to convince myself during those moments when I felt like running that a little should be OK. In hindsight, I really didn't know better. Here's where I learned that the push to go back to my old ways just wasn't worth it. My one last hoorah:

One night after work, I went to the gym and got on the treadmill. I made a mental note of the woman on the machine next to me. I was 31, she was in her 40s. I looked at my pace on the treadmill, then I looked at her pace on her treadmill screen. She was older and running faster. That's when my competitive nature kicked in.

Deranged me kept hitting the "speed up" button on my treadmill until I was outpacing her. I was going to show her! (As if she really cared, I'm sure.)

Man, did it feel good! Well... until it didn't. I suddenly felt lightheaded. I felt an intense rush through my body with the sensation of my breath being taken away. And then it happened.

This part of the story was retold to me by another gym-goer: I passed out. I was catapulted off the back of the treadmill. I smashed into the mirror behind me. And I was promptly taken to the emergency room.

Oops. That was a dumb move!

This is when I finally admitted to myself that running and intense exercise really were not worth it anymore. This is when I wholeheartedly took my own medicine; I began walking, doing yoga, and helping others whom I thought could benefit from learning from my experiences.

That experience at the gym was when I started my 20+ year journey as a volunteer and spokesperson for the American Heart Association.

This was an amazing way to channel my experiences and put my energies into advocating for other people, particularly women, who don't necessarily stand up for themselves and their own health. There is something so gratifying about speaking with a woman one-on-one after one of my group presentations.

So often, people would tell me how they had felt like something was wrong, but they either didn't act on it, or they had gone to a doctor who gave them a similar brush-off I had received years earlier.

Here's what it sounded like:

"Oh, it's probably that time of the month."

"You could be dehydrated."

"You likely had too much caffeine."

"You're stressed because you're a mom."

After hearing this, I would always say, "I'm not a doctor. I will not diagnose you. But from my own experience, and I highly recommend you go back to your doctor, or to a different doctor, and go with this list of questions; tell them A, B, and C; listen to your gut and don't wrap up that appointment until you feel satisfied with your answers."

Very often, I would receive an email or a call after that speaking engagement from the person saying, "I went to the doctor, and they found something wrong. I can't thank you enough." That fueled my realization that what I was doing *did* matter, and that my experiences could help other people.

One of the other key perspectives I gained and found really interesting, was people's reaction to my condition and what I had been through recently. Anytime I said the word heart, people freaked out. Rightly so. It is kind of an important organ. But I also realized very quickly that I had a disease that was controllable — not curable, and unfortunately progressive — but controllable. I had great medical care. I had my defibrillator. I had medicine.

I had finally come to the right mental conclusion to realize what I should and shouldn't be doing physically, such as: not getting thrown from a moving treadmill. I was able to live a relatively normal life. This really made me realize that I was so much better off than many other people. It gave me a real sense of empathy for people with late-stage cancer or for long-term debilitating diseases that hinder them from living a normal daily life.

This became another tool in my silver lining toolkit. I was not going to feel sorry for myself or let others put me in a damaged goods category. I realized a few months after my diagnosis that although this was the biggest thing in my life, I had to shift from being a heart patient who happened to enjoy a variety of things in life, to being a thriving young woman who happened to have a heart condition.

THAT was a huge, positive, life-altering mind shift. I did not let my disease define me. I let it fuel me. I had a zest for life and a desire to help others.

I definitely did not look like the poster child for heart disease, but I knew full well that this disease was only going to get worse over time. We didn't know what that timeframe looked like. And the outcome on the other end was likely going to be a heart transplant.

But until then, all I could do was tell myself that I had plenty of life to live between now and then. And it gave me a real opportunity to understand and feel for other people who were living through situations that were worse than mine.

This revelation started as a way to help other people prevent or get a handle on their heart disease. But in looking back now after 20 years, my mission was greater than that. I truly wanted to help people holistically. And although I didn't look at it in the organized fashion I do now, I've realized there are multiple dimensions of wellness that I embraced throughout my own life.

I hope to impart some of my life lessons to help others accept and adjust to their own situations.

So stick with me through a few more crazy stories and key learnings and we'll get to the meat of my Wellness Widget, which is my approach to a healthy and fulfilling life.

Chapter 3 – The Journey

ARE YOU READY TO go on a 20-year trip in one chapter? Sounds tedious, I know, but I promise if you bear with me, you'll be rewarded with some fun, suspense, education, and inspiration.

Close to two years after my near-death experience and my ARVC diagnosis, I woke up on the morning of September 11, 2001 like the rest of America, witnessing the tragedies unfolding across the US. It was obviously an exceptionally pivotal time in our history.

I was still living in the San Francisco Bay Area, which is an incredible melting pot of mostly transplants. Yes, some people actually grow up in San Francisco, but for the most part, people move there from all over the country, and all over the world, really. Within months, maybe even weeks, after the 9/11 attacks, much of my social network was moving back home.

When you live in a city full of people who are from somewhere else, and something like the magnitude of September 11 happens, people tend to gravitate toward what's comfortable — their family, their "home," their roots. I felt the same way, and as my friends were dispersing, I thought it was time to get back to Michigan.

I packed up my things in January of 2002 and moved from San Francisco to the middle of the country and started my next chapter. I grew up in Michigan. I had family and friends in Michigan. The company I worked for was headquartered in Michigan. It all made sense.

It made sense until that first road trip I made for work in a rear-wheel drive car in a snowstorm with a dead cell phone on I-75 while semi-trucks were whizzing past me. I white-knuckled it to stay on the road and finally made it home after eight hours, which should have been a four-hour trip. What was I thinking?

Welcome back to Michigan winter!

I bought a great little condominium, something I never could have afforded in California. I happily reestablished relationships with friends and family, and now was on the hunt for my new cardiologist. I found a wonderful electrophysiologist who specializes in arrhythmias, and although he wasn't super familiar with my rare disease, I was immediately impressed with his approach to my care and the connection we had.

I was also very grateful for how quickly he familiarized himself with the ins and outs of ARVC. After a couple of evaluations with Dr. Kim Man, we determined that it would make sense to perform a procedure that would eliminate some of the extremely fast arrhythmias and give me some relief from the imminent threat of overexertion turning into a dangerous heart rhythm.

Some of my ventricular tachycardia (v-tach) episodes would go as high as 280 to 300 beats per minute. Definitely uncomfortable and absolutely dangerous. Through a cardio ablation procedure which was recommended to me years earlier but never actually performed, he thought he could eliminate some, if not all, of these abnormal electrical impulse sites.

Allow me to explain v-tach. Take your two fists, right fist on top and left fist on the bottom, and squeeze them alternately. The right fist is your atrium (blood in) and your left fist is your ventricle (blood out). Keep squeezing alternately every second or so in even intervals, and that's how a normal heart beats.

When I go into v-tach, basically, my right ventricle takes over and starts beating exceptionally rapidly. The atrium can't keep up and whatever little bit of blood can seep in from the right atrium into my ventricle is what keeps me alive. When the heart rhythm is exceptionally fast (for me anything higher than 270 bpm), not enough blood can get through and I pass out.

Dr. Man's thinking was, find some of these overactive electrical sites and ablate them (burn them closed), and we could eliminate or certainly reduce the amount of fast tachycardia. Tachycardia can be deadly, and although I have a defibrillator to counteract the irregular beats, no device is foolproof. Eliminate the sites, reduce the risk.

I went in for my first ablation. (I have had several others since.) The medical team performed the procedure in a catheterization lab. They lightly sedated me, but I was awake and aware. They may at times have given me instructions to do certain things during the procedure, so I couldn't be "out." They numbed a spot in my groin with a local anesthetic, inserted a catheter and threaded it through a vein into my heart.

I distinctly remember the first catheter journey from my leg to my right ventricle. I felt this sudden and quick "zipping" through my body. I actually giggled. The giggle was a combination of the tickling sensation and my defense mechanism against feeling uneasy.

Once they were in my heart, they used adrenaline and electrical impulses to stimulate the diseased sites and simulate my fast v-tach. Once they found the spots, they ablated them, removed the catheter, and I was on my way. The procedure was quick and painless. In and out.

"Go home and rest for the remainder of the day," they told me.

I'm not very good at taking those kinds of instructions. I went home, took a nap, and within hours of my hospital visit, got up and went to the mall to buy a new outfit for a date I had the next night.

I found a cute little ensemble. *Hooray!*

Spoiler alert. My date never saw it. *Boohoo!*

As I was getting ready for (let's call him Ian) to pick me up on Saturday, I went downstairs to the lower level of my condominium to get my laundry. I ran up the stairs with my loaded clothes basket, and immediately went into v-tach. I guess they didn't get ALL of the diseased spots in my heart (and I likely didn't rest enough).

I made it to my bedroom, sat on my bed for a handful of minutes, hoping that my tachycardia would convert out on its own. I tried lying down, but the feeling of my 200-ish beat-per-minute heart rate felt so uncomfortable.

Lying back only exacerbated the feeling when my heart was pressed against the mattress. I sat back up and realized after about 10 minutes it was time to call 911.

Unbelievable! Ian was on his way to pick me up.

The EMT's strapped me in the gurney, hooked me up to all the machinery and monitoring equipment and loaded me (in my adorable new outfit) into the ambulance. Once the sirens were going and we were speeding toward the hospital, I asked the paramedics if I could have my phone so I could make a call:

"Hi! Uh, Ian? Yea, it's Kristy. The craziest thing is happening right now. I'm in the ambulance on the way to the hospital. I think I'm going to be a little delayed."

Seriously! I treated this call like my cat just threw up and I'd be a little late because I had to quickly shampoo the carpet.

I assumed his response would be a half-hearted, "Let's reschedule. Talk to you later. Bye." Then I'd never hear from him again. Instead, he actually asked:

"Which hospital? I'll be there within 30 minutes."

What?!?!?! This was only our third date. I didn't know how to process this. So sweet. Definitely awkward. A little extreme? *Whatever... let's just play it out and see how it goes*, I thought.

In the meantime, my heart was racing at 240 bpm, and I just wanted it to go back to normal. I would deal with the awkward relationship issues later.

I got to the hospital, and Dr. Man just happened to be on call, thankfully, so he met me in the ER, along with the Medtronic rep. Medtronic is the brand of defibrillator that was implanted in my chest when I was in San Francisco. The rep was the one who would actually manipulate the device.

"We're going to sedate you," they said. So I would be completely out.

They were going to change the settings on my device so it would shock my heart back into a normal rhythm. Just prior to inserting my IV for sedation, I looked up to see Ian. He was certainly a sight for sore eyes! No wonder he didn't want to call the date off. He looked good and surely didn't want to waste an opportunity to impress. The nurses certainly noticed.

Prior to applying the defibrillator pads, they needed to remove the gown from my upper body. I'll never forget the awkwardness: Dr. Man looking at me, looking at my date, looking at me and saying, "Is it OK that he sees you bare-chested?"

Briefly mortified, I giggled. "Sure. He's fine."

Then I was almost immediately out from the sedation. I woke back up in a normal rhythm, all went well, and Ian was very sweetly sitting by my side, holding my hand.

I spent the night in the hospital. Instead of ditching me for more interesting plans (like watching The Matrix for the fourteenth time), Ian went out and bought me a wonderful, healthy meal from Whole Foods accompanied by a book of poetry that he actually read to me bedside. He totally won over the nurses. Who brings their date poetry and reads to them in the hospital after having a cardiac incident? I'm guessing this didn't happen too often.

I was released the next day and was reminded how I should not be pushing myself when I get doctor's orders. This was a theme I seemed to be overlooking.

Fast forward a few months. I was continuing to go into v-tach. Not as fast, but sometimes for hours on end. After any episode longer than eight hours, I would take myself to the ER for another defibrillator manipulation. We finally figured out that one of my medications that was supposed to suppress arrhythmias was actually promoting them.

Meds work differently on different people, and this one was definitely not a match-made-in-heaven for this patient. Dr. Man researched options and fortunately found a cocktail of drugs, using an older medication that not many heart patients use. It was my miracle combination! It is common for patients to "break through" meds as their disease progresses, and prescriptions need to be changed out. I am happy to say this older drug was my stabilizer for almost 20 years. He really hit the nail on the head.

Within my first year of being back in Michigan, I became very active with the Heart Association.

I threw myself into all their major campaigns: the Heart Walk, the Heart Ball, and Go Red for Women when it launched in 2004. I had the opportunity to speak to large crowds of women and men about the impact of being proactive with your heart health. I "preached" how important it is to self-advocate with your doctors and for women to stop putting everyone and everything else ahead of themselves and take care of their own health.

If you haven't seen the Elizabeth Banks "Just A Little Heart Attack" video on YouTube, feel free to put this book down and watch the 3:14-minute clip. It is funny, poignant and memorable. And it undeniably illustrates how easy it is for women to worry about everything and everyone else except themselves.

Through the American Heart Association, not only was I humbled knowing that I was directly impacting people's behaviors and health outcomes, I was honored to meet and present with celebrity speakers like Star Jones, Rosie O'Donnell, Chris Powell, Susan Lucci, and others.

Eighty percent of heart disease is preventable through lifestyle adjustments. Being a promoter of this life-saving message — with high-profile heart health advocates and the American Heart Association staff — has provided some of the most rewarding times in my life.

Life was good — I was behaving and my heart was behaving. In 2004, I was at my company's annual conference. On the last night, we always had a big celebration. I was on the dance floor with several of my friends and was enticed to cut some serious rug with one of our Spanish colleagues who without a doubt knew his way around the dance floor.

As a reminder, my ARVC is exacerbated by elevated exercise (including dancing), and also by alcohol. I had learned that I could typically do one or the other, but combining the two doesn't usually result in a positive outcome. Here I was in a situation about to do both. Not one of my better judgment moments.

While Fernando was whipping me across the dance floor, endlessly spinning me around and flipping me over his back, I all of a sudden felt myself go into v-tach. I doubled over, gave him the Heisman, indicating that I needed him to cool his jets and back off.

Fortunately, a couple of my work friends saw me looking like I was in despair. They hurried over and two of them grabbed my elbows and walked me over to the closest flat surface, a nearby coffee table, and guided me to sit down.

At that point, I knew I was either going to pass out or get shocked. I did not pass out. Unfortunately, I was fully aware, as were my two friends, when my defibrillator earned its keep and shocked me. Not only did I feel like I had just been kicked in the chest by an angry horse, my friends said they felt remnants of the shock, too. They were still holding on to me when the 10 joules electrified my body.

I'm not quite sure who was more surprised — them or me. "Shocking" as this was for everyone, the good news is, my defibrillator did what it was supposed to do, and I was alive. I was back to a normal rhythm. I called it a night and retired to my hotel room. I was a good girl this time. Maybe five years into the fainting and shocking thing, I was finally starting to learn my lesson.

In July of 2004, my life took the best turn I could have ever imagined! Two years of working together, being great friends, watching each other in other relationships we secretly wished would fail, and yes — he saw the whole dance/shock thing go down at the work meeting earlier that year — timing finally worked in favor of my now-husband and me. We were both unattached during the summer of 2004 and jumped at the opportunity to "give us a try."

On our first date, we both knew we would get married, and he is now my partner for life. I am extremely proud to call him by his actual name, no alias. My amazing husband is Dave Sidlar. No trying to protect the innocent here. He's definitely guilty of stealing my heart! We were engaged in 2005 and married in 2006. He has been by my side through doctors' appointments, medical procedures, good news, bad news, and uncertain times. He continues to be my absolute rock (not to mention the funniest person I know)!

A variation on the Spanish dancer theme happened at our wedding reception. Oddly, this time with a French friend. What is it about these European dance magnets? My French friend is an exceptionally talented swing dancer. He requested one of his favorite tunes and pulled me onto the dance floor. We definitely drew a crowd; he's that good.

As much as the crowd was focused on his slick moves, their faces quickly shifted when they saw me back away, double over, put my hands on my hips, and stumble to the closest chair. I was sure I was going to pass out — at my own wedding reception! I sat down, and fortunately was able to convert out of my fast rhythm without having to embarrass myself by getting shocked in front of all my family and friends.

As if that weren't enough for one night. Dave and I left our reception and checked into our hotel room for our requisite wedding night activities. Dave being the funny guy that he is declared that it was no fair that our friend almost made my defibrillator go off by over-exerting me. That was now his mission. Could a night of bedroom Olympics cause me to get shocked and him to feel the electricity at the same time? Really?!?!?! That was what was on his mind on our wedding night. As we do, we laughed together about it. So, did he attain his goal?! Some things are best left to the imagination! Choose your own adventure.

In 2007, it became time for my ICD to be replaced. The battery usually lasts between four and eight years. Mine was at the eight-year mark. It really hadn't been put to the test as often as many other patients needed to rely on theirs. I was fortunate to get the full life out of mine before needing a replacement.

The second surgery was much simpler than the first. They made an incision on top of my existing scar, opened up "the pocket," took out the aging defibrillator, which is the size of a small pager, and replaced it with the new one. The device has a mechanism that looks like a phone jack (if you are old enough to have had a home phone and know what that looks like) that is attached to the leads (wires) that are threaded into my heart. After eight years, those leads are likely infused into my heart muscle and not coming out. The "jack" feature allows the medical team to unplug the old device and plug in the new one.

They stitched my incision, woke me up from my semi-lucid sedation and sent me to recovery. I was released from the hospital within an hour. Piece of cake. There isn't nearly as much recovery or pain as the first implant, but I still had to lay low for first couple of days. You'll be pleased to know I actually followed doctors' orders. Something about having a caring spouse who ensures I'm doing as I'm told might have something to do with that!

Over the years, I continued to have annual checkups, including regular echocardiograms. My first few years' reports always included statements about my enlarged right ventricle and thinning heart wall.

I got very used to seeing these words describing my most important organ. Within a few years, the reports changed to say *severely* enlarged, then ultimately *exceptionally* enlarged after about 19 years. This was part of the constant reminder that my disease was indeed progressive.

"Dr. Man, can I get a transplant?" I asked during every annual appointment.

I so badly wanted a new heart. I wanted one that worked like everybody else's. I was tired of not being able to push myself physically, and I was admittedly envious of my friends who were running 5Ks or joining fitness groups with intense workouts, and even of my mom who at 70-something ran a half marathon. I was tired of not being able to drink and dance when I was out with my friends. I was tired of having to stop when walking up a hill.

Dr. Man would just look at me in disbelief every year.

"Kristy, you don't want a heart transplant until you *need* a heart transplant," he always responded, "and you don't *need* a heart transplant yet."

This became an ongoing joke between us.

"Yes, things are getting worse," he would say, "but you're doing fine, and you just need be patient."

One milestone of me recognizing that my heart was indeed getting worse was when I traveled to Brazil for work. In a matter of three days, I spent 22 hours on planes — 11 hours down, a day of work in Sao Paulo, and 11 hours back. When I arrived home in Michigan, my feet were so swollen that they were literally being squeezed out of my shoes, and the exposed area was puffed out to at least twice the size. My ankles (if you could even distinguish that I had ankles) looked like those of an elephant. It was the first time I truly didn't recognize a part of my own body. I was disgusted and a bit freaked out.

It was late on a Friday when I called Dr. Man's office and spoke with the doctor on call. He asked me some questions to rule out blood clots and said, "You have edema from my insufficient heart function."

Between the flying, not moving enough, likely eating too much salt (confirmed–we had some amazing, well-seasoned Brazilian food), and probably not drinking enough water, it all added up. I was relieved, but it was also another indicator that I was getting worse. This was to be expected, but sometimes it was just a bit of a shock to the system actually hearing it.

I continued along, watching my sodium intake, drinking more water, and taking my medication combination, which was still working exactly the way we wanted it to. One day I went to refill my prescription, and they had discontinued my 200 mg dosage. It was an old medication that few patients were taking anymore, so they stopped manufacturing it — my miracle med.

Dave and I called multiple pharmacies and investigated how we could possibly get our hands on the 200 mg dosage that I needed. Upon consulting Dr. Google, we discovered that although fewer and fewer humans were taking Mexiletine, it was still a common drug for dogs. From that day forward, Dave started referring to my meds as my German Shepherd pills. I kid you not, at that moment, Dave asked me:

"Should I start calling around to veterinarians to see if we can get your prescription filled?"

It was funny at the time, but frustrating because I was on such a good path with my med combination. We ended up being able to make some adjustments with other dosages (instead of 200 mg x three per day, we did 250 mg in the morning and 150 mg at 3 in the afternoon and 11 at night).

All's well that ends well. *Woof!*

In 2014, I was asked to move to Singapore with my job. They wanted me to manage the sales team across the Asia Pacific region — China and India, down to Australia and New Zealand, and all of Asia in between. After much contemplation and excitement and conversations with my family and my cardiologist, we decided to accept the offer and make the move.

Dr. Man reassured me that some of the best medicine is practiced in Singapore. He would help me find a great doctor there. He was not concerned about me moving halfway around the world and was confident that my care would be very good. We made the decision and took the plunge!

I had one last task to complete before we moved–get that tattoo I had been dreaming about. I never thought of myself as the tattoo type, but promoting awareness about heart health and heart disease prevention had become such an integral part of whom I was becoming.

The Go Red for Women movement was critically important and very sentimental to me. If you aren't aware, the symbol for Go Red and women's heart health is a red dress. I wanted to get that symbol tattooed above my heart, over my defibrillator.

I got the OK from Dr. Man. The morning of my tattoo appointment, I did a little more internet research. It never dawned on me that the tattoo gun is magnetic and could set off my defibrillator. *Ooops.* I read conflicting reports (as one does when researching something on Google).

I went to the tattoo shop, and we decided to try it out by turning the gun on while hovering it over the left side of my chest. Success! No weird alarms or, God forbid, shocks! Ten minutes later, I was donning my new ink. I love it!

Side note: Due to trademark laws, I was not allowed to replicate my tattoo on my book cover. My illustrator replaced it with a cool heart-shaped design. I will be infusing this into my next tattoo!

Off to Singapore we went in March of 2015. My boss will never forgive me for expensing $7,000 to move my cats halfway across the world, but everything about that move equated to one of the best decisions Dave and I ever made. I could write an entire book on our three-year Asia experience, but for now I'll stay focused on my health and wellness journey.

We quickly settled into our amazing new city/state/country, and I set out to find a cardiologist through recommendations from multiple medical professionals. I was indeed very impressed.

Things were going very well in Singapore. My first six months were relatively uneventful from a heart perspective. It was very hot. Average annual temps range from about 80 to 90 degrees Fahrenheit with average humidity around 70%. Singapore is one degree from the equator, so the weather is perpetually tropical. We didn't have a car and walked most places, including the steep hill leading to our apartment. For the most part, I was trucking along — until Thanksgiving Day during our first year in Singapore.

As you can imagine, American Thanksgiving is not observed in Singapore, so I spent the day at work. I had a very busy schedule ending with a big client presentation. Leading up to the meeting, I forgot to take my medication. I also didn't make time to drink enough water. After the meeting, I had a glass (or maybe two) of champagne with my colleague. I went back to the office and finally left for home around 7:30 p.m.

I looked at my watch and realized I had three minutes to catch the next bus. I ran across the street, and because I had not properly taken care of myself that day (no meds and little water on top of now having alcohol and running – stupid, stupid, stupid), I went into v-tach on the sidewalk next to the bus stop. I felt myself going fast and ready to fall hard; I knew I was going to pass out.

I got myself as low to the ground as possible to try to reduce the distance between my head and the pavement. And sure enough, everything went dark. I woke up to a half-dozen Asian faces standing over me.

"Are you OK?" asked one nice man holding out a water bottle.

Of course, I knew what had happened. My heart rate had gotten above 250 beats per minute. I passed out. My defibrillator shocked me, and I came "back to life." Common practice for this American girl.

I got up, brushed myself off, straightened my skirt, got on the bus, and went home. I'm sure the crowd was in disbelief.

Dave was traveling that week; he was in the Philippines. When I got home, I called to tell him what happened. Yes, he was very caring and concerned, but I'd be lying if I didn't tell you that I got a bit of a scolding for not taking care of myself throughout the day. I hung up and everything hit me.

It's Thanksgiving. I'm halfway across the world. I'm by myself. I almost died (well not really, but I guess I could have). I got onto Facebook to see everyone posting pictures of their turkeys being prepped and their families all together enjoying their wonderful holiday with people they love, and here I was alone in my apartment in Singapore. Yes, at that moment I hosted a little self-pity party complete with a nice serving of salty tears. It was my first bout of homesickness, and admittedly a little bit of fear overtook me.

A few minutes of a good cry can make anyone feel better. Off to salvage Thanksgiving. No turkey dinner for me that night, but I did go into the kitchen and specifically chose the turkey-flavored cat food for my two felines. At least they got to enjoy a nice serving of poultry on the last Thursday of November in 2015.

A few days after my bus incident, I had to fly to China for work. I took an afternoon flight, got settled into my hotel room in Shanghai, ordered room service, hopped into bed, and fired up my laptop. I got a phone call, and as I was pulling my cell phone across my body up to my ear, my defibrillator alarm went off. If you've been to Europe or watched any of the Jason Bourne movies, you can likely conjure up the sound of a European ambulance siren. That was the sound emanating from my chest.

I didn't feel like I was in any kind of strange rhythm. I didn't feel off in any way. My first thought was that my cell phone triggered my defibrillator magnet (highly unlikely, but not completely out of the question). I assumed it was nothing, but then slight panic set in when my brain kicked into gear that maybe my new defibrillator (my third one that I had implanted right before moving to Singapore), could be faulty.

What if all of a sudden, out of the blue I get shocked? I wasn't mentally prepared for the horse-kicking again. All these things started going through my head. The alarm stopped after 10 seconds, and everything was right with the world. It was 9:05 p.m.

The next night, I was at dinner with colleagues in a relatively noisy restaurant. We were looking someone up on LinkedIn when, just like the night before, my defibrillator alarm went off. My Chinese colleagues looked at me with puzzled faces.

I was mortified, but was able to get creative and quickly came up with, "Wow! How strange! This guy has some crazy sound effect on his LinkedIn profile. I've never seen that before!"

I completely deflected the focus from what was actually going on inside of my chest. I looked at my watch and saw that it was 9:05 p.m., the same time as the night before. I deduced that something was triggering my defibrillator at the same time every day.

All of a sudden, it dawned on me that the next day I would be flying back to Singapore on a plane at 9:05 p.m. What would the nearby passengers think, when all of a sudden, the woman in 17C started beeping? What would you think? Perhaps that the woman has (or is) a bomb and is sitting next to you on a plane.

Holy shit! What was I going to do? I had to get home and I couldn't change my flight time at this point. I got on my flight as scheduled, and at 9:00 I got out of my seat, went to the lavatory, locked the door and stood there until 9:05 when my trusty defibrillator sung its song. After 10 seconds, I went back to my seat, as though December 5 on a plane from Shanghai was a day just like any other.

Obviously, something was wrong with my defibrillator and once I was home I needed to see my doctor. All I could think of, though, was how extremely busy my Friday work schedule was. I didn't have time to go to the doctor. Trying to sell this rationale to Dave led to the first time he had every raised his voice with me. When I told him that I would go on Monday because I was just too busy, he lost it!

"Goddammit, Kristy! You have got to go get this checked out! Your health is more important that your work."

That made me sit up straight. I cancelled a few meetings and went to the doctor. I learned something about my new defibrillator that day. It has a built-in mechanism that if when I get shocked or go into serious v-tach, I'm supposed to go to the doctor so they can check me out and turn off the alarm.

Who would think lying unconscious beside a bus stop and almost dying would be a reason to see your doctor? Jeez! OK...lesson learned!

The more I traveled, particularly during my last year-and-a-half in Asia, I noticed I was getting much more edema (swelling of my lower limbs). My cardiologist advised me to drink more water and eat less salt, particularly before I travel, but it was just part of heart failure and heart failure advancement.

We finished our three years in Singapore and moved back to our home in Michigan.

I had a car again and I would drive myself to work, parking in the back of the lot. There was a slight grade from where I parked to the front door, and I was noticing shortness of breath and fatigue while walking to the building. My first instinct was, "Oh no, my heart's getting worse." But then I thought maybe it could be something else; I was actually hoping it was something else.

I went to the doctor and learned through bloodwork that my B-12 was low and that could easily have been causing my fatigue. B-12 shots got my levels back to normal, but I was still having a hard time with some of the very basic exertions. We determined that indeed my heart failure was getting worse. That proved itself through a few other incidents.

My next validating moment was at a conference in San Diego. I was walking from my hotel room to the conference center. It was probably a quarter-mile walk with a slight grade. At this stage of my heart failure, my mind had started noticing (and lamenting) every little grade in my path. I knew it was going to mean discomfort, especially if I were in a situation where I had to walk *and* talk at the same time. My stamina just wasn't what it used to be.

"Kristy!" someone called as I was walking.

Shit! Someone wants to walk with me to the building… and talk… and I'm carrying my heavy (well heavy for me) briefcase. This is going to be fun.

I met up with my client, and after about one minute of walking and talking, I had to ask her if we could stop. I was so embarrassed.

"I have a health issue and need a break," I said.

She was very kind and understanding, but it was definitely one of those smack-in-the-face moments that reminded me that things were getting worse.

I was also noticing with greater frequency that wheeling my suitcase through airports, especially if there was any grade, could stop me in my tracks. I would have to pull off to the side to catch my breath, sometimes multiple times, between my gate and the Uber. It was frustrating to say the least.

And then there was our Yellowstone National Park trip in June of 2019. We had been flyfishing for a few days and eating like kings and queens at the lodge, probably consuming way too much sodium and more wine than I should have. Being at altitude didn't help, and I'd be surprised if I consumed enough water in between all the fish we were catching! I honestly felt like hell the day we were in the park. Although most of the day was spent in the car looking at the sights, we did get out several times to take in the scenery up close.

I remember one pivotal instance when we walked from the parking lot up a walkway to a waterfall. I probably had to stop six times in a distance that would have normally taken me less than five minutes. I felt like I had a football in my gut; this was a new sensation for me. I wasn't quite sure what was wrong, but it was very uncomfortable and very frustrating.

We got back to the car and my phone rang. It was Dr. Man calling with my most recent echocardiogram results. This was the time that my report went from *severely* enlarged to *exceptionally* enlarged, and for the first time in our almost 20-year relationship, I noticed Dr. Man expressing some real concern. He gave me recommendations around how much sodium to consume, what foods to avoid, and how to measure sodium intake. Fortunately, I was not much of a salt eater (sweets have always been my downfall), but 1500 mg of sodium a day is an aggressive goal. I was up for the challenge.

When I got back from Yellowstone, I had a more probing conversation with Dr. Man.

"It's time for you to be referred to an advanced heart failure and heart transplant specialist," he said, going into sales mode: "His name is Dr. Lanfear. He's a really great guy. You will love him. He is so nice. He's really great with patient care. He is such a good guy."

I finally stopped him. Of course, I was grateful to know that I would be working with someone who would treat me well, but assuming this was the guy who was going to put someone else's heart into my chest, the words I was craving were competent, accomplished, and successful, to name a few.

"It's great to know he's a nice guy," I said, "but is he good at what he does?"

"Absolutely," Dr. Man said.

Coincidentally, I put two and two together and figured out that Dr. David Lanfear is the brother of a friend of mine. We had actually met at a party a few years ago. And yes, indeed, he was very nice. And I now know that he is also extremely skilled at what he does.

Dave and I met Dr. Lanfear at his office, I explained the football in my gut, and he validated that a distended liver is a common sign of advanced heart failure. The first level of congestive heart failure is fluid retention in the limbs, which I had been experiencing for a few years at this point. With advanced heart failure, the inefficiency of a diseased heart doesn't allow for proper blood flow through all the central organs, causing back-up and discomfort, particularly in the liver.

I was again reminded about sodium intake; I assured him I was adhering to my limit. He also gave me a new water intake threshold of 45 to 50 ounces per day. That was less than I had gotten used to. With advanced heart failure, too much water can lead to more retention, swelling, and strain on the heart. I actually had to back off on my intake. At that time, I truly became addicted to my Apple Watch, and particularly my WaterMinder app.

The appointment concluded with him telling us that it was time to start really keeping a close eye on my progression and that a transplant would likely be in the near future. But whether the near future meant six months or several years, no one knew.

Chapter 4 – The Progression

LIFE GOES ON, BUT this part of my life was taking some major twists and turns–both personally and medically. Dave and I had been planning a move to California part-time. We went through the process of looking for, and ultimately buying, a house in the Oakland Hills, outside of San Francisco. We knew this was not ideal from a medical care perspective, but we knew we could make it work. Between tele-medicine and planning my doctor appointments around other trips back to Michigan, we would be fine.

We found our (near) perfect house. We absolutely fell in love with the setting, the layout, the views, the location, and the charm. They all outweighed the one less-than-desirable feature when looking at it through the eyes of a heart failure patient. It has 47 steps from the front door leading up to the driveway at street level where we park our car.

Yep, every time we left the house, I would count every one of those 47 steps. Only twice in six months did I make it all the way to the top without stopping. And there were those not-so-infrequent occasions, especially in the beginning, when we would realize after getting up to the car that we forgot our sunglasses or our bridge toll pass or our water bottles.

Dammit! That meant one of us (thankfully, usually Dave) going back down 47 stairs and back up 47 stairs — huffing and puffing even harder after round two. We love the house and location so much! It has all been well worth it.

Usually the 47 steps weren't so bad, because we would park the car at street level, and when we had to carry heavy things — like from shopping at Costco or coming home from the airport with our suitcases — it was all downhill, not bad at all.

But my worst memory of those stairs was when I left the house at 6 a.m. to catch a flight. It was dark. I was traveling for a full week, so I had a very heavy suitcase, not just to carry-on. It must have taken me close to five minutes to walk up those 47 steps, stopping multiple times, grunting, sweating, finally reaching the top, so frustrated with my body, pouring myself into the Uber and having to hold back the tears from spilling past my lower eyelids. Of course I managed. The trip was fine. And I looked forward to coming back home where walking down the 47 steps was a whole lot easier.

COVID hit in March of 2020. We had planned to come back to Michigan anyway in May. And the assumption was that we would be back in the fall, after enjoying six months in the lovely Michigan summer. We reached home on May 8 and had an appointment with Dr. Lanfear a few days later.

After my examination, when I gave him some feedback on how I had been feeling for the last six months, he said it was time to formally begin evaluating me for heart transplant. In *my mind,* evaluation meant, *let's go through some testing and see if I actually need a heart transplant at this time.* In his mind, it was a little closer to being time to transplant me, but we needed to go through the full evaluation before we could get me on the list. I eventually had to reconcile this in my own head.

First of all, the evaluation process is very intense. They take you through every test imaginable—not just cardiology tests, of which there are A LOT—but every other medical test. They would put in orders for a colonoscopy, mammogram, dentist appointment, bone density, pulmonary function, every blood test under the sun, dermatology, and immunizations (heart transplant recipients can't have live vaccines after their immune systems are suppressed post-surgery).

I had sessions with a psychologist and social worker, and I would ultimately meet the surgeon (whom I later found out was someone other than Dr. Lanfear). The thought behind all of this testing is that they don't want to give a new, healthy heart to someone who could potentially die of cancer or some other serious illness, or be mentally unfit to take care of a new heart and the new challenges that lifestyle brings.

I had been dreaming about a heart transplant for longer than a decade. But all of a sudden, I was battling with this volley in my head, *I'm still relatively healthy. Should I try for more time on this side of a transplant? Knowing that the average life expectancy after a transplant is 12 to 15 years, where does the greater benefit lie? Do I want to fix this now and get a better quality of life sooner, or do I risk shortening my life on the other end, because of how many additional years my transplant may give me?*

Some people don't make it to the 12- or 15-year mark, while I know people who have lived 25 and 30 years post-transplant. This was such a battle in my mind.

But here was the part about being on the list that was really messing with my head. Once I was on the list, every day could be THE DAY. This inspired me to tick down a mental check-list of what I needed if I were suddenly called into surgery.

"Did I shave today?" Getting stuck in the hospital with hairy legs sounded mortifying.

"Did I get all my documentation into our systems at work?" Well, of course not. I'm a salesperson. We hate documentation.

"Did I tell everyone I love them?" Fortunately I was pretty darn good about that, even before transplant was on the horizon.

The other bummer was that I wasn't allowed to be more than four hours from the hospital at any given time. Thankfully, it was COVID and there wasn't much traveling happening, but assuming I could be on the list for months (or years?) this could really cramp my style.

Speaking of cramping my style, I want to take a little departure from the obvious symptoms and downsides of having heart failure and looking transplant in the mouth. This football in my gut thing was a really tough part of me living with heart failure. Sure—it was a constant reminder that I was getting worse and that my general, day-to-day health was declining, but here's where it really got me.

I had serious body image issues. I suffered from it most of my life—anorexia in college, exercise bulimia in my early 30's, serious anxiety about having my picture taken in a bikini, which meant letting people see my body minimally clothed. Plus, I hated people touching my stomach (as in I could have a cock-my-arm-back-and-want-to-hit-someone feeling if someone touched my mid-section). I of course wouldn't really have hurt anyone, but it was a serious aversion that lived with me for decades. I wouldn't say it was debilitating, but it was a constant mental battle.

And now with my distended liver, I would look at what *had been* my favorite body part—my flat stomach—and be near tears seeing this bulge under my right ribcage. I could no longer wear clingy tops. I had made the awful (in my own mind) switch to a one-piece for the first time since I was probably 15, and it got so bad I didn't even want Dave to see or touch me anywhere around my stomach. This was really fucking with my head. As much as I hated it, the upside was that it drove me to want to fix it.

So, we agreed to start the process and see what everything looked like after evaluating my test results. My evaluation took almost five months. This was a combination of things: with my more-than-full-time job, it was difficult to get to all my appointments without having to take an inordinate amount of time off. I spread them out and tried to schedule early and late-day appointments, which was not always easy to do.

Throughout my appointments and evaluations, I kept hearing the same thing from new doctors, techs, and nurses: "Really? You? You don't look like you need a heart transplant. You would never know looking at you. You look so healthy."

These comments kept fueling my fire, thinking that I was still a ways off from actually receiving a new heart. As much as I wanted a new lease on life, I have to admit the reality of it all was starting to feel pretty daunting.

Here was something I found really interesting. During one of my visits, Dr. Lanfear described that amongst the many types of advanced heart failure, left-sided heart failure (which is trouble mainly in or starting from the left ventricle) is by far most common. Isolated right-sided heart failure — what I had — was not so common.

According to data from the European Society of Cardiology, right-sided heart failure only accounts for 2.2% of heart failure hospital admissions. Of course, I couldn't be common, right? Left-sided heart failure is better understood in how the symptoms manifest and the rates of progression–usually more steadily over a period of time. And there are also better-established ways of gauging risk.

Right-sided heart failure can progress quite differently, and there is a lot less knowledge about how best to estimate risk.

Add that I had ARVC, which threw in additional arrhythmia risk, and made my right-sided heart failure even more unpredictable. I could be doing just fine, then without warning I could just "fall off a cliff," as Dr. Lanfear put it. I heard him, but I don't really think I "heard" him. My testing continued.

One evening when I was at a friend's house, the most unexpected thing happened. I was sitting at her kitchen island when the European ambulance siren went off inside my chest.

What? How could this be? I hadn't had a v-tach episode and certainly hadn't been shocked recently (or at all since that lovely episode at the bus stop in Singapore). I couldn't figure out the reason for the alarm. But since I learned my lesson in China when I didn't get my device checked, I made an appointment the next day to get it evaluated.

The device nurse draped the magnetic reader over my ICD as I waited for some benign update such as, "There was an upgrade to the technology," or "Your battery is warning us that it's in the last 24 months before having to replace it." Either would have been fine, and as for the latter, I would likely be getting a transplant before the battery died, so who cared?

Then the nurse asked, "What were you doing Monday morning at 6:45 a.m.?"

"Sleeping," I answered.

"Sleeping? No way! You got shocked!"

OK, remember I told you that getting shocked by my device was like getting kicked in the chest by a horse? There is NO WAY I got shocked while I was sleeping. I will admit I'm a super solid sleeper (makes Dave jealous since he only gets about an hour of deep sleep a night), but trust me–I would know if I got shocked.

Unless...

All the previous times I hadn't remembered getting shocked were the times my heart arrhythmia was so fast that I passed out. It was all making sense now. I remembered waking up that night with a sharp pain in my side. That was the sensation when my ICD delivered a mild pacing to settle down my rapid rhythm. Apparently, that pacing made my heart jump to one of my ultra-fast v-tach arrhythmias and I passed out in bed.

I realized that Dave must have been in one of his rare moments of deep sleep. He never felt the bed shake when my body convulsed from the shock. At the same time, another piece of the puzzle started to fall into place. One of my cats had been afraid to sleep on the bed with me the rest of the week. We couldn't figure it out. He was such a nighttime cuddler. I bet he was laying on or near me when I got shocked and he either was so startled by my intense, sudden movement, or he actually felt the joules because he was touching me.

This was a lot to take in! Why would I just randomly go into v-tach with zero exertion? *Um...stress, you dummy!* My husband and I, who both worked for the same company, were both let go the previous Friday during a round of COVID-related cuts. That would cause a bit of stress, don't you think?

One of my most memorable experiences during my pre-transplant evaluation was my final echocardiogram. The seasoned echo tech was teaching a cardiology fellow how to conduct the test. She applied the ultrasound goo to my chest and placed the rollerball thingy over my heart. She maneuvered around for a while capturing images. She would occasionally call the experienced tech over to review her work. Just as he sat back down at his monitor for the fifth time, the fellow proclaimed that she was really having a hard time finding my right ventricle.

"It's there," I assured her. "I promise you. And not only is it there, it is REALLY hard to miss!"

By this point, remember, my right ventricle was categorized as *exceptionally* enlarged. Moments later, and this is when I realized that the young fellow was still learning the art of bedside manner, she announced, "Holy moly! That thing is HUGE!"

I refrained from actually saying, "I told you so," but we had a good laugh.

By the end of my exam, we established that my new ejection fraction (EF) was 27%, well below the normal range of 50% to 70%. Ejection fraction measures the amount of blood pumped out of the heart as compared to the amount of blood contained within the heart. A lower percentage indicates lower heart function. Forty percent EF is the baseline for heart failure. I was certainly not as low as some, but clearly within the scope of heart failure. No surprise, just a numerical validation.

During my meeting with the surgeon, it became very clear that when getting a new heart, you trade one set of problems for another. Fluid retention goes away, shortness of breath goes away, and the daily threat of death goes away (this was a pretty compelling argument).

The other side of the transplant comes with medication-induced risks of: cancer, diabetes, kidney problems, high blood pressure, increased cholesterol.

All this on top of constant vigilance to ensure I didn't reject the new heart.

Wow! He wasn't kidding. Was being able to run again worth all this?!?!

During that appointment, he also talked a bit about right-sided heart failure and its sudden rapid progression.

"When was the last time was you got shocked?" he asked.

Really?!?! He is asking me this just weeks after that crazy sleeping episode? Had I met him last month, I could have confidently said it has been at least five years. I had to 'fess up (and admit to myself), that I had a recent episode. He validated that this was likely an indication that things were getting worse.

This brought us near the end of my evaluations, to the point at which the Heart Transplant team would present my case and determine if I would go on the list or not. The team at Henry Ford Health System consists of more than 20 medical professionals who meet every Wednesday and review whichever cases are up for a decision. Five of the team members had met me face to face. There were 15 other members in the room who knew me only by what was included in my ever-growing medical chart.

By all accounts from the five people who had actually laid eyes on me over the last few months, although my tests were showing the severity of my heart failure, I still looked healthy, was exercising regularly, albeit at a lower intensity level, and felt relatively fine.

The people on the team who had never seen me before were not able to compare my medical records to how I actually looked, which as I had been told, I did not look like a typical pre-heart transplant recipient.

Based on my records and the results of my extensive evaluation, the team, hands down, said, "This patient needs to be on the list."

One team member, Dr. Lanfear later told me, chimed in with, "I don't know how this woman is even able to walk down the hall by herself. Her heart is grossly enlarged." He said they rarely see a right ventricle that looks this bad.

Later that morning, December 1, was the official day that Dr. Lanfear made the recommendation that I go on the list. I suddenly had a litany of questions:

How long will I be out of work?

"Usually three to four months. Give yourself the time to heal. Recovery is not a quick process."

Three to four months felt like an eternity.

Will I be able to run again?

"Most patients are able to go back to the physical activity they enjoyed prior to heart failure."

This was absolute music to my ears!

When can I get on a plane again and start traveling?

"Let's evaluate it at six months. Your immune system will be really fragile, and we can't have you in compromising situations for the first six months. The first year is when we have to watch you most closely."

Six months is do-able.

What about receiving "the call"?

"You need to stay within four hours of the hospital at all times. We will call you; we will call Dave; and after two attempts each, the transplant coordinator will have to move on to the next candidate on the list. Basically answer any phone call that starts with the 313 area code!"

No travel more than four hours away? What if this takes a year? That sucks. No escapes to California? Huge bummer, but OK. Again, all worth it.

I had such mixed emotions when we hung up: excitement knowing that I was going to be given a new lease on life; anxiety that once I was on the list I could get the call any day (was I really ever ready?); pissed because I was discouraged to fly out to California for our family get-together due to my fragile medical state and the increase in COVID cases during holiday travel.

My dad and stepmom, Linda, had been planning our Christmas gathering for months. My brother, Marty, Dave, and I were to spend five days together at their house in northern California. We hadn't *all* been together for close to a year, and I hadn't seen Dad and Linda since April, eight months prior.

One of my doctors was a little less strict and said ultimately the decision was up to me. It was very possible to stay safe while traveling by air. Cases were increasing in California and hospital beds were becoming scarce. That could have become a real risk if I contracted the virus.

Another cardiologist called me later that afternoon practically in tears, begging me not to get on a plane.

"It's way too risky!" he said.

I've come this far. What if I were to get COVID because of plane travel?

"I'm nearly certain you would not survive if you got sick in California where ICU beds are limited," the cardiologist said.

Our plans had to be put on hold. The family understood, of course, but it was such a sad day and really a tearful decision. On top of all this commotion and emotion, the reality was starting to sink in that this transplant was imminent. This was for real. My life, my family's life, and the life of some unsuspecting person and their family, were about to change forever.

Chapter 5 – The Reality

WE HAD A WONDERFUL Michigan family Christmas full of traditions, great food, gratitude, and the bittersweet reminder of why we were missing some family members in person. COVID kept too many of our relatives at home in other states. Zoom calls had to suffice so we could bring Florida, California, Arizona, and Michigan together in one "room."

After enjoying that fabulous, restful, social week between December 25 and January 1, it was time to start making plans for my transplant listing. This is when I just about gave Dr. Lanfear his own heart attack. Here's how the call went:

Dr. L: "Let's set up an appointment for you to get officially listed. Can you come in next Tuesday?"

Me: "Well. I was thinking. I've only been in this job a couple months. I just hired five new people. I have a big sales kick-off meeting (virtual) set for January 19. I'd like to wait until after that."

Dr. L: *silence, maybe some eye rolling, maybe some inner-voice swearing, surely some self-talk to remain calm and not yell at his patient.*

Me: "Is that OK?"

Dr. L: "Kristen...

Me: *Oh, God. He addressed me by my formal name. I think I'm in trouble.*

Dr. Lanfear finally became audible and explained that as a medical institution that has formally approved me for a heart transplant, which no one does lightly, they could be responsible if something were to happen to me. He was telling me I was ill enough to be listed, but my election to wait was not lining up with that logic. If I fell off that cliff he described earlier, we could all be in a dire situation.

We had a friendly debate around the topic. I am a salesperson after all, and have spent my whole career negotiating. I persuaded him that waiting a few more weeks would be OK.

My sales kickoff meeting went off without a hitch. I was happy, and now it was time.

At this point, I was battling with whether or not to tell my employer. I had only been with The Mom Project — a digital marketplace that helps moms get jobs — for four months. I was about to get a new boss. How would she feel about me announcing that in any number of months, I could be taking three or four months off to recuperate? What if she were one of those leaders who was going to come in and clean house and bring in her own teams? I had no idea if my transplant announcement could be her excuse to "manage me out of the business."

I had this debate over and over in my head; I talked to a close friend who is an esteemed HR and benefits leader. Dave and I debated the merits and pitfalls of both sides.

"Nice me" wanted to be up front. Everyone else said that I was not obligated to tell anyone, and to let the transplant timing play out on its own. This was very difficult advice to accept, but in my brain, I made it make sense. Could you imaging me sharing the news, being let go, and not having a job with insurance? Having a multi-six-figure surgery, not to mention the additional multi-six-figure claims post-surgery for however many months and no way to pay for it? The thought gives me shivers.

Within days of my last conversation with Dr. Lanfear, my nurse called and said, "So we have one more test you need to do. No big deal. Can you pop into your lab and get a TB test? After that, we'll be good to go, and you'll be on the list."

I was a compliant patient (this time). The tuberculosis test for transplant recipients isn't the common skin test. It is a whole-blood test that indicates, through a white blood cell reaction to antigens, whether or not TB is or was present.

Three days later, after my blood did its thing in the petri dish, my nurse called and said, "You're not going to believe this, but you have TB. Well, latent TB. Somewhere along the line, you contracted it."

I did live in Asia and Mexico for extended periods of time, so it seemed plausible.

"You have a strong immune system," the nurse said, "so you never got any of the symptoms, but the bacteria are still in your system. We have to get rid of it before we can do a transplant."

Just when I thought I was ready to roll, here comes a setback. Of course, my mind went to wishing I would have just said yes to Dr. Lanfear in early January. Something told me he did, too! *Oh well, we are where we are. Let's just roll with it.*

Right after my TB diagnosis, I met with a senior infectious disease doctor at the hospital. He did an amazing job explaining latent TB. Many people have it. I had probably lived with it for years. As a normal, heathy person with a strong immune system, it is not a big deal. However, after my transplant knocked my immune system back to virtually nothing, I would have a very high risk of actually suffering from TB. Basically, it could finally rear its ugly head.

There were two avenues of treatment for latent TB. He mentioned the first one — three months of antibiotics. I couldn't believe what I was hearing, having to take pills for three months and possibly not being able to get on the transplant list. I was bummed, but accepted the news, knowing there was no way around the treatment. He followed this explanation with, "This three-month treatment might interact with the variety of heart meds you're already taking. I'll need to check."

He left the room for a few moments to research any contra-indications with my current drug regimen. He came back into the exam room and said, "Yes. Your mexiletine is on the list. There is a drug metabolism issue, so we cannot put you on the three-month course. We'll have to go with the other treatment." I was thrilled to think maybe it would be something a little bit more rapid.

Oh no! Did I hear him right? Did he just say...

"The alternate treatment that is best for you is nine months long."

What?! All of the sudden I felt a boxing match of thoughts pounding through my head.

Fortunately, this only meant a short delay in listing me. They would put me on the antibiotics for a month and ensure that I was doing OK, and at that point they could put me on the list.

Back to my struggle about telling my boss. I was still being pulled toward giving her some kind of heads-up. I felt like I needed a way to give her and many others at The Mom Project a peek into this heart world I've lived in for 20 years. I wanted them to get to know me a bit more, and give our CEO, other leaders, and my employees a way to see why heart health is so important to me. I wanted them to get a feel for why I have been such a passionate women's heart health advocate over these last couple decades. And as always, I hoped it would impact some of the people who may have never thought about examining their heart health history, or their eating habits, or their other wellness factors like stress, sleep, water consumption, et cetera.

The universe was in my corner. Because of my strong affiliation with the American Heart Association, and as the sitting chair of the Detroit board, I was contacted by a local Detroit news station and interviewed about my heart history. It was a three-minute and 40-second version of the first four chapters of this book. They played the segment on National Wear Red Day and posted a written version with a video link on their website and other social media outlets. This was my cue. I immediately sent it to my boss in an email, texted our CEO, and posted the video link in our company social media channel.

What a relief. It was out there. I received heartfelt, encouraging comments. There was a genuine interest in how I was doing, and they seemed truly grateful for my advocacy of women's heart health. After all, women are the heart of our company's mission.

I was very careful in my news piece to say, "I will need a heart transplant *someday*." No way was I going to say publicly that I would be on the list in a matter of weeks. Although being on the list didn't guarantee me anything. It would likely be months or possibly over a year before I would get "the call."

By now, a month had passed since my infectious disease appointment with Dr. Alangaden. We met again at the 30-day mark, 11% of the way through completion of my nine-month TB treatment. Everything was in order. This was early March of 2021. We were finally ready to get on the transplant wagon. Everyone was in agreement. No negotiating. No push-back. Just ready. Really ready! All of us!

Dr. Lanfear set up my appointment for March 10, 2021. On that day, I would officially be listed with UNOS, United Network for

Organ Sharing. UNOS is a private, non-profit, scientific, and educational organization that administers the only organ procurement and transplant network in the U.S. You may know of other organizations–Gift of Life, Donate Life, and LifeShare, for example. These organizations support UNOS nationally through local organ recovery programs. I was so close to being a part of their great work. This was finally happening!

Chapter 6 – The Cliff

As I WAS LOOKING forward to that March 10 appointment, my body decided to remind me of that conversation I had with Dr. Lanfear several months ago — the one about right-sided heart failure, and particularly ARVC, being less predictable and not typical like left heart failure.

March 5 was a Friday, and that night while I was sleeping, I went into ventricular tachycardia. I didn't think much of it the couple times I woke up. My heart was aflutter, and it was bothersome, so I checked my Apple Watch a few times, saw that the rate wasn't all that fast, and fell back asleep. When I woke up on Saturday morning, it was still noticeable. The annoying part about my v-tach this time was that it was fast enough to feel abnormal, but too slow for my defibrillator to kick in and help me.

So, I just continued to feel this uncomfortable, spastic feeling in my chest. I paged the on-call nurse and was told that there really wasn't much they could do over the weekend and to come in on Monday morning to get an EKG. This may sound like negligence, but that's the beauty of having a defibrillator. As long as it was functioning properly, it would keep me safe.

I went through the weekend in a slow but uncomfortable arrhythmia. My heart rate was hovering somewhere between 75 and 90 beats per minute. That may sound like most people's normal heart rate, but my resting heart rate was usually around 45 to 50. And unlike a heart that is beating normally, mine was beating primarily using only my ventricle, not that steady atrium ventricle pattern I described earlier.

Friends noticed that I was a little lethargic. I wasn't quite myself, and my energy was definitely turned down a notch, but I (gently) powered through the weekend. I laid low, treated myself to a mani/pedi, and was really looking forward to getting to the doctor on Monday morning. After 58 hours in v-tach, it was finally time to get back to normal.

Dave drove me to the cardiologists' office first thing in the morning after completing a few work meetings first. *Cue his eye rolling.* Dr. Man wasn't in the office that day, but one of his partners was. He said he would see me right away. As we were walking from the parking lot into the office, I felt an intense sensation, like I might suddenly lose my footing–not quite at the passing out stage, but I knew my heart rate went even more haywire at that moment.

I immediately slumped over and sat on the ground. I could feel my rapid heart rate now close to doubling what it was a few minutes before. I was too weak to walk, so Dave got a wheelchair.

As soon as he came back, I felt like I was having a hypoglycemia attack, so he ran into the little market in the medical building lobby. He got me a couple hard-boiled eggs. That always did the trick. I ate one-and-a-half of them. I had no energy to finish the second one. I just wanted my heart to start beating normally and pumping blood through my body. It needed proper energy.

Dave wheeled me into the cardiology office. I was slumped over in the chair as he checked me in. I had very little energy, I felt really crummy, and I just wanted to lie down. They got me into the exam room as soon as they could and got me up on the table.

I was hoping it would feel like a relief to be horizontal versus putting energy into staying upright in the chair. But as soon as I got on the table, since I was lying on a relatively hard surface and my back was pressed against the table, all I could feel was that fast flutter inside my chest.

The nurse took my EKG, and the doctor came in moments later. He looked at me. He looked at Dave. After a brief explanation of the rhythm he was detecting on the report, he said:

"You need to get to the ER...now!"

Fortunately, the ER is right across the street. Dave wheeled me back downstairs and parked me in front of the building while he ran to get the car. I very unsteadily folded myself into the car, fumbled with the seatbelt, gave up and banked on the fact that Dave could get us a quarter-mile in one piece.

He dropped me off at the ER receiving area. A nurse wheeled me to the triage area. Dave parked the car. This next part is a little foggy because I was so drained of any clear ability to think. Blood was not pumping the way it should and it was affecting my ability to focus. Yet suddenly my focus was very clear. I needed something to throw up into.

"Nurse! Help please! I'm going to be si — "

She got there just in time with the mauve-colored, kidney-shaped dish which I dutifully filled. The eggs. They were what my body needed at the time, but now, not so much. With my little pink plastic receptacle still at the ready, just in case, they wheeled me back into an ER room. Dave arrived just as they were parking my gurney.

To my good fortune, Dr. Man was at the hospital doing rounds that day. He was there! Best news of the morning! Once they checked my vitals (and I was actually starting to feel a little more normal), they wheeled me into a nice, private room. Dr. Man came to see us and explained that he had called the Medtronic rep who would soon be able to manipulate my defibrillator and get me out of this awful rhythm.

As soon as all parties were present, an IV was inserted, the "good juice" was flowing, and I was properly sedated so they could shock my heart back to a normal rhythm. When I came to, I was A) happy to see Dave's sweet face; and B) even happier to feel so much more normal. More normal, but not perfectly normal like all the other times they had shocked me. I still felt a little off, and my heart was still fluttering a bit.

I found out later that Dr. Man, behind the scenes, was calling Dr. Lanfear and coordinating my transfer from this hospital to the hospital where my transplant team was, about 20 miles away.

This was my Cliff.

I got into the ambulance while Dave drove down on his own. My ambulance driver and his partner, the one who was in the back with me, were hysterical. Because I love a good conversation and I am a naturally curious person, I decided to pass the time with a little Q&A.

"Have either of you guys ever felt the shock of an ICD?" I asked.

They proudly started telling me stories about how they often practiced procedures on each other. They had inserted IVs, drawn blood, and strapped immobility devices on each other. We were all laughing as they recounted some of the situations and inside bets they had made with each other to see who could tolerate more pain. They did admit they had been tempted to test the defibrillator, but thought better of actually trying to shock each other. "Good move," I said, with a look of extreme caution. "You're much better off not knowing what you're missing." And I again used my horse-kicking analogy.

The stories and conversation kept us occupied until we arrived at my ICU room at Henry Ford Hospital in Detroit.

"Thank you, guys! I wish you well," I said, adding playfully, "and I hope I never see you again. Keep the shock paddles in the case when you're around each other!"

It was 8 p.m. on the 8th of March. I settled in, said goodnight to Dave, went to sleep, and waited for orders the next day.

On Tuesday morning, nurses came and went, taking my vitals, drawing blood, and giving me heparin shots in my stomach to prevent clots. Without fail, any time my feet were peeping out of the bed-sheets, a nurse would comment, "Oh! your toes look so pretty!" Dave rolled his eyes every time.

One of the transplant doctors came in and told me that they would be able to get me on the list that day. Hooray! I was planning to be on it the next day anyway, since I had a previously scheduled appointment with Dr. Lanfear on March 10th. My situation was now considered critical. They wanted to act now!

The transplant list rankings are very well defined. Here is my very layperson's explanation:

- Level 1: critical, non-dischargeable, ventilated, life threatening arrythmia.

- Level 2: non-dischargeable, either needing a heart pumping assist device or in ventricular fibrillation or tachycardia (**ME!**).

- Level 3: not having to be in the hospital, but either needing a portable heart assist device and/or a myriad of other advanced heart failure issues.

- Level 4: heart failure confirmed but stable (**this is the level they planned to have me at if I hadn't had my v-tach episode that led me to the ICU**).

- Level 5: waiting for multiple organ transplants.

- Level 6: All remaining active candidates.

I was listed as Level 2. This status was very familiar to me. My close friend's brother had had a heart transplant four months earlier. He was very sick. He was a Level 2. He got a heart in two days. I was not nearly as sick, but I could still hope for a quick call!

I asked my nurse, "Now that I'm in the hospital and at a Level 2, how long do I stay here to wait for a heart? What if it takes weeks? Do I just hang here the whole time?" The thought was mortifying. *I might die of boredom first.*

She responded with, "One of the patients down the hall was here for three months before receiving a heart. He was level 2. Pretty toes!"

My worst nightmare was staring me in the face with a real-life example just down the hall a few rooms away. I could not fathom the idea of sitting in the hospital for three months waiting for my heart. The alternative would be leaving the hospital and being bumped down to a Level 4. And then who knew how long I would have to wait?

Ay yay yay. What a crazy juxtaposition. Nothing I could do about it, but wait it out and see what happened. And hope I could be like my friend's brother — Level 2, two days.

Once my listing was official, I alerted my manager and told her that my transplant was now imminent. It felt great to have everything out in the open. She was amazingly supportive, and my conversation with her further validated The Mom Project's incredible people, culture, and encouragement of their employees when the unpredictable happens.

I channeled my hospital boredom into wrapping up all my outstanding work and creating a transition plan for the time I would be out. Dave sat patiently by my hospital bedside. He brought me lunch and dinner and we had a typical, fun day together. The surroundings weren't ideal, but we found ways to bring light into the day.

Dave headed out at the end of visiting hours. He made a few calls to friends and family. On his drive home, he called to tell me about one of them. This remains my all-time favorite, sweetest story from the pre- and post-transplant phase of my journey. Our "niece" (our dear friends' nine-year-old daughter) had asked her mom very seriously and somewhat anxiously:

"Mom, will Aunt Kristy's new heart still love Uncle Dave?"

Seriously?!?! How absolutely adorable, and special, and insightful, and naïve. It absolutely melted my heart. Still does every time I think about it. Keep reading to learn the answer to her question.

My project for the next day was creating Facebook and text groups so Dave could communicate with everyone while I was in surgery. I asked him if I could give him my phone and let him use that to keep everyone informed. I set up a family group, a work group, a college friends group, a local friends group, and a random-all-over-the-place friends group. I also started a dedicated Facebook page called "The Transplant Tribune: Kristy's Getting a New Heart" and invited about 150 people whom I thought would want to stay up to date on my journey. They invited several others and I think the list grew close to 200.

It was nearing the end of visiting hours–8 p.m. on Wednesday night — and Dave was preparing to go home. As he was shoveling his things into his backpack, we talked about how cool it would be, although unlikely, if someone would come to my room that night with the good news of a heart. We were allowed to hope, right?

Just as he leaned over to kiss me goodnight, my mobile phone rang. It was a Detroit number, but not the hospital prefix. I looked at it and set my phone down, since I was enjoying our little moment. I said, "It's a Detroit number, but not the hospital. If it was good news, someone would come tell me in person, right? I'm here in the hospital."

He gave me that look and said, "Why don't you answer it? You never know." I slid the bar on my iPhone and said, "Hello, this is Kristen." (My formal name is what was on all my hospital records and what everyone on the team called me).

The woman on the other line said, "Hello, Kristen. We have some good news. We are calling to let you know we have a heart for you!"

Wow... I am tearing up as I write this. It was such an incredible, indescribable moment.

I was literally fist-pumping with infinite joy while I fumbled to put the phone on speaker so Dave could listen. I had a smile from ear to ear. Dave and I exchanged smiles and tears and nervous glances. I kept my composure the whole time I was on the phone as they were explaining next steps, who would be in touch next, and how I would be wheeled down to the OR at 4:30 a.m. But I could not stop thinking about the fact that the last 20 years of having a shit heart were coming to an end, and I was about to have a new path for my life.

Dave and I hugged and cried and took the obligatory hospital bed, pre-transplant selfie. I wanted to memorialize the moment, but I also wanted to post it on my Facebook Transplant Tribune to let everyone know that we were officially on our way to Kristy 2.0 (my favorite term coined by a good friend of ours).

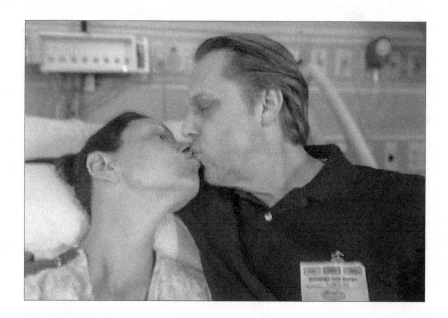

As soon as Dave left, I called my mom and her significant other, Richard; I called my dad and stepmom, Linda; and I called my brother, Marty. Dave was doing the same thing with his family from the car on the way home from the hospital. I knew everyone was processing this in their own way, but my hope was that my absolute excitement as I was sharing the news would ease their anxiety a bit. I acknowledged that everyone was able to feel what they were going to feel, but that I was calm, happy, and truly eager (versus anxious) for what was to come the next morning.

Dave went home. Just about as soon as he crossed the threshold of my room, the nurses got busy. They were like bees in a hive getting prepared for my 4:30 wheel-out in the morning. I can barely remember all that they were doing, but of course, one of them commented on my pedi. They drew blood, administered pre-surgery pills and shots, performed EKGs and other monitoring, and shaved my bikini line in the event that they couldn't insert the heart catheter in my neck and had to go through a vein in my groin.

Right after I got off the call, I assumed I would not be able to sleep because my mind would be all over the map. But after the flutter of activity by the nurse staff, I was pretty worn out. It was now about 1 a.m. As soon as they were done, they shut the door, I turned off my light, and was asleep in minutes.

I found out later that Dave went home and promptly poured himself a bourbon on the rocks. Don't judge. This was a lot for him to deal with. I think we all felt like things were a bit out of our control, and we all dealt with that the best we could. The harsh reality for Dave, and I'm sure the rest of my friends and family, was *what if I were to die?* He would be left behind. They would all be left behind.

I hate to be so harsh, but the very limited amount of time I thought about the possibility, and it truly was only a couple times, I wouldn't know any different. I hated that my family would worry while I was in surgery, and I certainly didn't even want to give thought to me not making it through, but I suppose there was always a small chance. If a stiff drink and some time to calm his own racing mind were what Dave needed, I'm glad he found his perfect distraction before drifting off to sleep.

He later told me his sleep was more restless than mine. Among several factors, I'm sure, was that his reliance was on an alarm clock and an iPhone. If he overslept, he would never forgive himself. There was no chance I was going to be late to my own surgery, so that factor was eliminated from the equation for me. I slept like a baby.

Dave showed up promptly at 3:30 a.m. He crawled in my hospital bed for a bit while we snuggled, and laughed, and hugged, and kissed, and assured each other that this was going to be the greatest day of my life. Literally, this *was* my life!

They were supposed to pick me up at 4:30 a.m., but came in shortly before that to say the heart was delayed due to weather. It would likely be closer to 5:30. We didn't know where it was coming from, but it was on a helicopter or a plane.

Here is something I learned about organ procurement when I was going through the pre-transplant evaluation process. There are two surgeons on the transplant team. One surgeon stays at the hospital and helps to prepare for the transplantation itself. The other surgeon goes to the donor heart for a full examination. They perform all the typical cardiac tests I had been through. In my case, the tests were always to see how bad my heart was. In this case, it was just the opposite; they wanted to see how healthy the donor heart was.

The two surgeons converse about the state of the donor heart, they transmit images, they review test results for HIV, hepatitis, CMV (I'll tell you more about that little virus later), they review any health risks the donor might be passing on (had they ever taken illicit drugs, or had any other social habits that could pose problems once transferred to my own body). At the end of their evaluation, the decision was made. This was a GREAT heart for me.

Another thing I learned during my pre-transplant education was that a transplant patient can be brought into the operating room, completely prepped, sedated and ready to go, only to realize that the heart (either from the virtual review or once it gets to the recipient's hospital) should not be transplanted. Something makes the surgeons uncomfortable. They pull the prospective recipient out of sedation thinking he or she has a new heart, only to realize that's not how things went down because the heart wasn't a match. Thankfully, this did not happen to me.

At 5:30, the nurse and a handful of the OR staff came to get me. Dave walked beside my gurney. There was some small talk with the staff, a little nervous chatter, and, of course, Dave's usual sense of humor and unmatched ability to make people laugh were in top form.

When we arrived at the OR doors, we said our goodbyes, and we told each other we loved each other. This was it! I had a genuine smile on my face. Dave had one too, but to this day I truly don't know what was going on behind his seemingly happy expression. I feel like Dave was trying to shield his anxiety, but we both knew I was going to be just fine and the surgery was going to turn out exactly the way we wanted it to.

This may be hard to believe, but I had zero fear, zero anxiety — nothing but positive thoughts about what life was going to be like on the other side. Again, I still worried about my family being worried for the next eight to 12 hours while I was under the knife. And I definitely was not looking forward to recovery. But dammit! I was getting a new heart and nothing made me happier!

We got me settled into the operating room. Super bright lights, cold room — I asked for a few additional blankets. They brought me nice, warm ones. They had some good music playing. The staff was chipper and amiable, and they occasionally included me in some general chatty conversation.

Then they got very focused on the serious stuff. They inserted a line into my arm that required absolute steady hands on their part and zero movement on mine. They taped my arm to a board to ensure nothing moved and used an ultrasound to find the exact location and angle of the vein.

Meanwhile, unbeknownst to me at the time, my mom from Florida and Dave from the hospital hallway were both on the internet, scanning The Weather Channel app on their phones, looking to see where there were storms. They both wanted know where this heart was coming from. Of course there was curiosity, but it's not like them knowing the location would have filled in any other blanks for them. How old was the donor? Male or female? What tragedy led to my wife's/daughter's life being saved today? I honestly think it was more a matter of giving them something to do other than worry.

While my medical team was working away, the anesthesiologist asked me if I had any questions. I had been asking questions for days (well decades, really) and felt so prepared for this. There was really nothing left to ask. So with a big grin, I looked at the anesthesiologist and said,

"I actually do have one more question. Michigan or Michigan State?"

He looked as though I had just asked him that one question from his medical school exams that he perpetually dreaded. The one that always used to stump him in school. There was genuine panic on his face. I could see his wheels turning while he was likely thinking:

If she's a Michigan fan and I say Michigan State, she could lose her faith in me.

Or maybe he just had that look because he thought I was the craziest patient he had ever dealt with. I like to think I was the most fun!

He grinned and slyly, slowly responded with,

"Ohio State."

We both laughed. *Well done, sir.* If I could have moved my arm I would have given him a fist bump. He knew he was in the clear.

And then they said, "Kristen, we're about to sedate you. Start counting back from 100."

And then...

It went dark.

Chapter 7 – The Transplant

Enter Dave for this part of the story. I certainly can't contribute anything interesting at this point.

Dave watched my gurney slip into the OR. His last glimpse of me was that really sexy hair cap they made me put on. My head was the last thing to disappear through the doors. Such a letdown of a memory to hold him over for the next who-knows-how-many hours!

The nurses shared with Dave how the day would unfold and what the cadence of his updates would be. She confirmed that the surgery typically took anywhere from eight to 12 hours. They assured him he would be contacted roughly every two hours. One of the nurses who was in the OR with me would call him from the room where she had a front-row seat. The first call would be when the heart was in the room.

The nurse headed toward the OR, and Dave's waiting began.

Since that day, I have asked him several times how he felt. Was he nervous? Was he scared? His answer is always, "You were good, so I was good." I honestly believe him.

Dave made an about-face and walked down the long, sterile hall to the waiting room. He sat in the waiting area with about a dozen other family members of patients going through a variety of surgical procedures. It was now time for Dave to get to work. He had updating to do. He grabbed both of our phones and started texting away to our pre-established groups. He would craft the first message–usually to one of our families — then copy and paste. He would sometimes modify the message slightly to fit the personalities of the other populations. Seven in total, plus the Facebook group.

I have since gone back to look through the messages and I can only imagine how the notifications function was working overtime from those two devices. Every time he sent something from his phone or mine, he was immediately flooded with a like, or a love, or a thumbs up, or the two exclamation points along with many comments.

He sent his first note to say that I had just been wheeled into the OR. He would check back in a couple hours. People responded:

"Thank you for the update, Dave."

"You guys are in our prayers."

"She's got this!"

"All the good vibes heading your way."

And the emojis were coming in fast and furious: prayer hands, the strong arm, every color of heart, thumbs up, fingers crossed, the smiley face with the floating hearts. You name it, they were steadily rolling in from all our amazing friends and families.

One of my favorite early responses from one of my lovely colleagues was, "Thanks, Dave!!! I'm on pins and needles over here, so I can only imagine how you're feeling."

Yes, people were supportive of me, but this was the time to pull out all the stops to support Dave. I still can't fathom how challenging this wait was for him, my family, and all the other bystanders! I'm still so glad I got to sleep through all the anxiety and waiting.

Dave stayed in the waiting room. After his first report-out to the masses, he settled in and got on social media to pass the time.

He scrolled through Facebook and Instagram, read a few car forums, looked at eBay to see what hot rods and trucks were on the market, and watched a few cat videos. He was getting a little tired of sitting, so he made his first move. He got up to buy something out of the vending machine.

Right on time, at the two-hour mark, he got his first call.

At 8:41, he sent his first update – short and sweet:

> First update from the OR nurse —so far so good. No issues. Prep was going well.

He put on a podcast this time for a little levity. He stayed put in the waiting area. Less than two hours later, he got the next call.

At 10:17, he sent update #2:

> The heart is in the room and being installed (I couldn't think of a better way to put it ☺). All is going well.

Dave is a car guy. The verb that came to his mind to describe this incredibly complex medical procedure was "installed!" Not transplanted, not implanted, not inserted. Installed! I think this post got the most commentary of any that day.

Dave managed the back-and-forth of the texts, then went back to his podcasts.

At 11:30, one of our dear friends called and said she was driving to the hospital and bringing Dave lunch. She was not allowed in the hospital, so Dave walked down to meet her. They shared a long, mutually supportive hug. There were no tears, just a strong under-standing that they were there to support each other and me.

They ate outside. Dave devoured his favorite — a Panera salad, half a sandwich, and a Chocolate Chipper cookie. They enjoyed good, comfortable conversation.

Around noon, now five-and-a-half hours into my surgery, he started feeling antsy about being away from the waiting room. He admits now that it didn't matter where he was; he was going to get the call whether he was standing in front of the hospital or sitting in the waiting room. Logic aside, he didn't like being away and was starting to feel worried since he was outside. He abruptly wrapped things up with our friend, gave her another hug and headed back upstairs.

He had barely been back in his waiting room seat when he got the next call.

At 12:26, he sent update #3:

> The installation process is still ongoing and all is well!☺

This message only went to a handful of people because less than 10 minutes later, Dr. Hassan Nemeh, my surgeon came out. He gave Dave the best news ever! I was just about wrapped up (or sewn up, as the case may be).

"The only thing that was remarkable was that there wasn't any-thing remarkable," Dr. Nemeh said.

The other surgeon, the one who flew to pick up my heart, was rejoining my breast bone with small wires and reconnecting my skin with surgical tape. They told Dave they would bring me up to ICU, but that it would be a few hours before he could see me.

At 12:35, Dave sent out update #4:

> The doctor just came out to talk to me and everything is wrapping up. She did great and there was nothing of note that came up during the surgery. The new heart is performing well and she will be moved to ICU in an hour or so and I will head up there.

His text was followed by heart emojis. What relief he must have felt.

Dave was truly AMAZING about ensuring no one went too long without an update. He was so great about making sure everyone would feel as much a part of the process as he did.

Dave sat for another few hours. This was when he discovered reels on Instagram. He was properly entertained until he realized that it was close to 3:00 and no one had called him to come up to ICU. He took the initiative and bid goodbye to the waiting room he never wanted to spend time in again.

He went up to the ICU floor, approached the nurses' stand, and asked what room. He felt a weird mix of curiosity and anxiety. He truly didn't know what to expect. He walked over to my room. The sliding glass door was open, the curtain was pulled, and he heard voices and movement.

Dave announced himself. One of the three nurses motioned for him to enter. He looked at her as he was talking, then immediately turned his eyes toward me.

Holy fuck! That was his first thought. His second thought was: *I am so glad Kristy's mom isn't here. This would have been brutal for her to see.*

He looked at me first, then scanned over to the IV machine. He was shocked to see how many lines. As he absorbed the mass number of them, his eyes traveled back to me, and that's when he took in the three drainage tubes coming out of my chest and the big central line in my neck. Everything either had something flowing into or out of it.

He looked back up at my face. Something was wrong. My lower lip was noticeably enlarged. And my tongue was hanging out of the other side of my mouth. It was being pushed out by the ventilator.

The nurse practitioner had noticed my fat lip as well. He examined it. No one had a confident explanation for it, but the assumption was that between the breathing tube or the anesthesia mouth guard, I bit my lip. Obviously pretty hard and for a LONG time.

Dave grabbed a chair and sat down at the end of the bed. He put his hand on my ankle while all the nurses tended to me at the head of the bed. Shortly after Dave sat down with me, Dr. Nemeh came in and was giving very specific instructions to the nurses about adjusting my med levels, monitoring my heart rate, increasing and decreasing certain fluids.

Dave said it was fascinating to watch the nurses' respect for his authority: "Yes, Dr. Nemeh."

"Right away, Dr. Nemeh."

"Of course, Dr. Nemeh."

He was in the room for about five minutes.

While everyone was tending to me, Dave thought this would be a good time to fulfill a promise he made to me months before. I had asked him, shortly after I knew I was going to get a transplant, if he would take a picture of me as soon as he first saw me. I wanted to see what I looked like coming out of surgery. Dave was trying to do this without anyone noticing. The last thing he wanted was for people to think he was some jerk of a husband who wanted something to hold over his wife's head later. After several attempts and almost-hads, he got the picture.

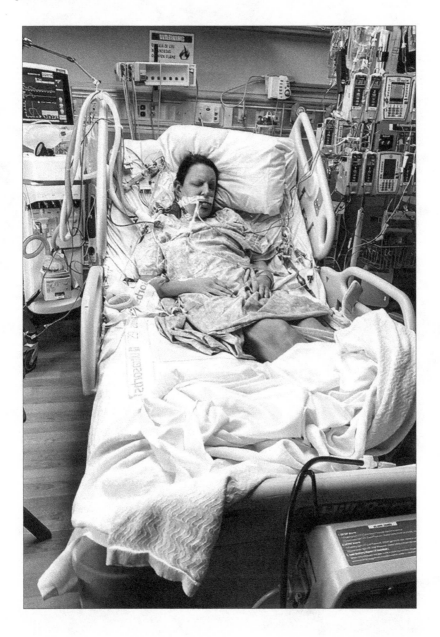

Chapter 8 – The Re-entry

AT 3:45, THE NURSE practitioner came in and announced that they were going to remove my breathing tube. He gently shook my shoulder to wake me up.

I'm back! I can take over from here...

(Well, I actually still needed Dave for the next couple days; I was more out of it than I was alert during the first 72 hours.)

Hearing what was about to take place, Dave stepped into the hallway. As he put it, "There are some things I just don't need to see." They needed me to be alert for the removal, since I had to follow instructions around inhaling and exhaling. I don't remember the actual removal, but apparently it was a smooth process. Moments later, they called Dave back into the room.

I remember feeling really hot. I started waving my hand, open palm toward my face. Apparently only I knew that I was trying to fan myself. Dave thought I wanted to hold his hand. He took it, and I complied only to release it a couple minutes later, waving it toward my face again. Dave grabbed it a second time.

I don't think I tolerated it for very long this time and weakly eked out, "I'm hot." They pulled the blanket off my feet. Dave felt dejected, I'm sure.

Right after they relieved my first bit of discomfort, I needed to let them know I had another problem we needed to deal with. I had a ton of gunk in my throat, and I was having a hard time swallowing and breathing. I was actually starting to feel a little panicky. I made the signal for wanting to write something down. My air pen was drawing something illegible in the air. They grabbed a pen and pad of paper and handed it to me.

With my eyes barely open, I wrote the letters p h l e m. Dave chuckled. Stories were later told how only I–the spelling and grammar chief of police–would actually know that the word for "gunk in my throat" is spelled with a "ph." He would have taken the easy way out and spelled it FLEM. For those of you who do know how to properly spell the word, I was mortified a couple weeks later when Dave showed me that piece of paper, which he saved. The correct spelling of the word is phlegm. I forgot the "g." Darn it, I was so close! I will forever defend my actions with the excuse that I was still under the influence of anesthesia. The doc instructed me how to clear my throat and I nodded back off.

At 4:35, Dave sent the last update of the day, update #5:

> They removed her breathing tube. She is breathing on her own. I kept hearing all the over-achiever things, best chest x-ray post-op, she's doing remarkable.

Overachiever! That word has been used to describe me a time or two in my life. Let me give you a tiny glimpse into my competitive spirit and how I'm motivated. Rewind to the psychologist appointment that was required as part of my transplant work-up. These appointments are critical to the evaluation. I mentioned earlier that they don't want to give a precious donated heart to someone who has a terminal illness or some other kind of physical indicator that they are not a suitable recipient. The same holds true with a patient's psychological health. I was asked questions from five categories:

1. Cognitive function — a lower rating could indicate an inability to maintain proper self-care post-transplant.

2. Adherence — heart transplant requires serious attention to taking medications on time, making doctor appointments, daily monitoring of blood pressure, blood sugar, weight, heart rate and many other things.

3. Mental wellness — a lower score could indicate making unhealthy lifestyle choices, like poor diet or inactivity, and having other psychological issues like depression or anxiety that could decrease survival rates post-transplant.

4. Social support — if I didn't have a supportive group surrounding me, it could lead to less positive outcomes.

5. Substance abuse — there are many physical risks to transplant recovery when the patient is over-using alcohol, drugs and tobacco, including other organ failure or worse, death.

Although I think I may have calculated 247 + 85 - 12 wrong on the cognitive test, I passed everything with flying colors.

Here's when the overachiever part of the conversation bubbled up. When the psychologist was asking me about how often I missed my meds (I had been taking seven pills a day for almost 20 years), I told her rarely, but that yes, I did forget on occasion. The psychologist raised an eyebrow and quickly launched into how critical it was that as a heart recipient I take all my drugs as instructed. She was very serious.

"You need to be an 'A' patient," she said.

Dave chimed in and spoke directly to the psychologist. "If you ever want to motivate Kristy to do what you need her to do, just tell her she's being a C patient. It will about kill her."

Never was a truer statement made about how I am motivated. The thought of a doctor telling me I'm "**that**" patient made me cringe. I'm a rule follower, I'm a star student, I do what's expected, and then some. I'm an overachiever when given the chance.

We were nearing the last few hours of Dave's visiting hours. I asked him recently how he spent his time while in my ICU room and I was just lying there. He explained that there was no time to do anything but chase nurses down. He said I was incredibly uncomfortable and about every seven minutes he was out in the hall trying to get someone's attention.

Barely audible, I would say, "I'm uncomfortable."

Dave would get the nurse. She would rearrange my pillows, and I would go back to sleep.

I would wake up and in a soft, but whiny voice, say, "I'm uncomfortable."

Two nurses would come in, lift me slightly, and place me in a seemingly comfortable position, and I would go back to sleep.

I would wake up and in a low, gruff voice say, "I'm uncomfortable."

Dave would go get the nurse again. She would shift my position and I would go back to sleep.

I would wake up and in a cranky tone say, "I'm uncomfortable."

One time, it took two nurse to lift me while Dave pulled the bed sheet up and created a comfortable (even if temporary) environment for me to rest. I fell back asleep.

At seven-minute intervals for two hours, that translates into this cycle happening roughly 15 times. No wonder Dave had no time to do anything else. I was squirmy; I was fitful; I was restless; I was being a pain.

Speaking of pain, during one of the nurse visits, she asked me on a scale of one to 10 what my pain levels was. I said, "I hurt a little–maybe a two."

I never remember being in actual pain, but man, I just couldn't get comfortable. Dave sat at my bedside and held my hand when he wasn't traipsing down the hall trying to find someone to ease my discomfort.

The nurses booted him out around 7:30 p.m. He had been up since 2:30 that morning and was feeling the weight and significance of the day. He wasn't tired as much as he was mentally spent. He kissed me on the forehead and headed toward the hospital garage.

As he was driving home, he called my mom. It was the first time he'd actually spoken to anyone by phone since I came out of surgery. He recounted more detail of the events that took place between his text messages. She hung on his every word. She was appreciative for the detail, but Dave said she definitely sounded worried. Of course she would! He picked up on her sensitivity and tempered the level of detail he shared. For example, he told her I wasn't very comfortable; he didn't recount the dozen-plus times he left the room to track down the nurses to relieve my perceived agony.

At 11 that night, Dave made a call to the nurse to get any last updates before he went to bed. She said my blood pressure was slightly elevated, so they adjusted my meds. Nothing else of note to report.

They told Dave I was comfortable enough to sleep. I'm guessing they "lied" to Dave just like he shielded my mom from the whole truth.

Day One was in the books. Dave went to bed and slept like a rock.

At 9:01 a.m. on Friday, Day 2, Dave sent his morning update:

> Morning update. I talked to her nurse around 11 last night and she was good. Her BP was a tick high so they adjusted her meds a bit. They gave her a little more pain killer and she was comfortable enough to sleep. I'm heading back down at 10 when visiting hours start.

On Friday morning, Day 2, Dave started his new arrival ritual–bringing baked goods for the nurses. His opening act was a variety of huge, fresh muffins from our go-to local bakery. He quickly became their new favorite visitor! After passing off the bag to one of the nurses who had been adjusting something on my IV monitor, Dave kissed me on the forehead. Much to his pleasure, I immediately smiled, focused in on him and said, "Hi, Love!" Maybe not quite with the level of enthusiasm he was used to, but he was happy to hear it, groggy voice and all.

Shortly after Dave settled in, another doctor came in to look at my still fat lip. There was concern that the swelling might be spreading to the rest of my face, and that would have meant something more serious. The doc patted and kneaded my cheeks, not seeing anything concerning. He pulled my lower lip out and down and saw the contusion. He concluded that the ventilator tube and my bottom teeth created a vice over my lip for six-and-a-half hours.

Dave looked on my hospital bed table and saw a bundle of toiletries in one of those little pink kidney-shaped containers. Yep, like the one I puked my hard-boiled egg into a few days earlier in the emergency room. In it was a tube of lip balm. He handed it to me and said it might make me feel better. I clumsily grabbed it and fumbled to remove the lid. That little tube became my addiction the entire time I was in the hospital. Instant relief. I must have gone through at least two tubes during my recovery.

A little before noon, the cheerful food service worker entered my room with my lunch tray. I swear they teach them to be extra enthusiastic when bringing in meals. Whatever it takes to lessen the disappointment when the patient lifts the covers off the plates of food. It was always such a letdown.

EVERYTHING about my Henry Ford hospital experience was fabulous. Everything except the food. It was truly HORRIBLE! If anyone reading this has any influence over the food services department at Henry Ford Health System, please take a picture of this paragraph and go make a difference! Before she left, she commented on my pretty toes and my nails. This was by far the most mileage I had ever gotten out of a single mani/pedi!

Even in my drugged-up state, I was able to distinguish tasty from virtually inedible, so Dave walked down to the lobby market and got me a chicken dish. That led to this additional mid-day post to a handful of people:

At 2:23 pm on Friday, Day 2, he sent this update:

> She has been moved to eating solid food. She had a little bit of chicken. It was actually quite cute. She would take a little bite of chicken and fall asleep for a couple minutes, wake up and repeat. She is doing well.

As the day went on, now close to 24 hours since Dave first saw me, I was becoming a little more alert. We had some conversations, albeit quite simple ones. He said my questions were very repetitive:

"When did I first notice you?"

"How long was my surgery?"

"What was the first thing I said to you?"

"Did you contact our families?"

Duh! As if he wouldn't have!

"When did they take my ventilator out?"

All these questions were asked between two and 10 times over the course of the first few days. He was Husband of the Year answering them as though I were asking them for the first time. Well, that's not the only reason he was Husband of the Year!

The next bit of post-surgery excitement was removing my catheter. I remember very little about the process. They said they were going to pull it out, and then it was out. Anticlimactic, but now I had a new set of freedoms: being able to go to the bathroom like a normal human.

Well, a tethered human. Every time I got out of bed, it took one to two nurses to untangle my three chest tubes, blood pressure cuff, IV lines in both arms (so many IV lines), the central line in my neck, and occasionally the cord from the device that housed my nurse call button. Even though I was able to walk to the portable commode by myself, a nurse had to carry the receptacle that captured all the fluid still draining from my chest tubes. Gross, I know. I tried not to look at the cloudy pink fluid slowly moving through the quarter-inch, slightly opaque plastic tubes.

At 4:54, on Friday, Day 2, Dave sent another update:

> Early evening update: Kristy is still doing well. She decided that the bed was a little uncomfortable so she asked to be moved to the chair. All of her vitals are good and she had a couple of good naps.

Dave's account of me wanting to move: I was restless and getting a bit whiny (he used the word grousing), saying once again that I was uncomfortable. The nurses actually prefer to move their patients to different positions, so they thought this was a good time to get me to move. As they approached the bed and started to scoop me up, they saw what a tangled mess I was with all my IV's and wires and tubes. I was like the meatball buried in a plate of spaghetti. Based on what they were looking at, there was not enough collective patience in the room to untangle me.

One nurse decided he was going to unplug everything and reconnect me. WAY easier. Once they had me all hooked up again, they elevated the back of the bed so I was sitting upright. I swung my legs over, and two nurses put their forearms under my armpits to get me upright. As soon as I was standing, one nurse wheeled my IV machine to follow my movement, one nurse bore the majority of my weight, a third nurse carried my drainage box, and I used all my strength to make the four steps from my bed to the chair. I made it and was sitting comfortably. *Aaaaah!*

At 8:15 p.m., Day 2, Dave sent his final update:

> Short update: Kristy is status quo. She was still in the chair when I left and starting to get a bit uncomfortable so I'm sure they moved her to the bed. She is a champ!

They did move me back. I slept well.

Dave called my mom on his drive home, and he, too, slept well for a second night in a row.

At 10:33 a.m. on Saturday, Day 3, Dave sent his morning update:

> Morning update. She had a good night. They are starting to wean her off some of the meds and her numbers look great. The surgeon was just in. They are going to take a couple of the drainage tubes out. They will leave one that he thinks will come out tomorrow along with the central line in her neck. She has moved from the bed to the chair again and as expected a little uncomfortable.

Shortly after Dave sent that text, the nurse practitioner interrupted my dozing to tell me that they were going to take out two of the drainage tubes in my chest. I was excited, because it meant two fewer things for me to get tangled in when getting out of bed or going to the bathroom. I heard him say something about morphine.

Wait! Don't they give morphine when something is painful? What was about to happen?

The NP described the removal process:

"First, take a deep breath in. Hold it. On the count of three, exhale. We will pull the tubes during your exhale."

Hang on! This is far too much instruction for my mushy brain to sort through.

This is how the conversation played out:

Me: "Can you say that again, please?"

NP: "Take a deep breath in. Hold it. On the count of three, long exhale. We will pull the tube while you're exhaling."

Me: "Hang on. I'm sorry. When do I exhale?" I was scared I would do something wrong and really pay for it. This seemed kind of important.

NP: "It's OK. We can take our time. You're going to take a deep breath in. Hold it. Then on the count of three, you'll exhale."

Me: "Can we do a practice?"

NP: "Of course."

Me: *Inhale. Hold. One, two...*

"Wait. Wait. I don't think I understand. I'm not sure when to hold it.

Can we do another practice? Will you say it again?"

NP: "Of course we can. Take a deep breath in. Hold it. On the count of three, exhale slowly."

Dave was standing in the hallway. At this point, his hand was covering his brow and he was shaking his head, rolling his eyes, and chuckling to himself.

Me: "I need one more practice, please."

Dave: *Oh my gosh. Kristy, you're embarrassing the family.*

NP: "OK. Take a deep breath in. Hold it. On the count of three, exhale."

Me: "OK. I'm ready." I was totally still convincing myself of that. *Let's just get this over with.*

NP: "Great. Let's go. Take a deep breath in. Good! Hold it. That's it. One, two, three, long exhale."

I don't remember feeling them pull the tube out and have absolutely no recollection of them closing up the hole with surgical tape. That all took a few minutes. I think I might have dozed off again.

The NP got me to wake back up and said, "OK. You did so well with that first one. We're going to do the second one now."

Great!

"Remember — inhale, hold it, slow exhale."

Oh my God. It's like I was hearing this for the first time. I had to ask the NP to walk me through it all over again. I will spare you the lines and lines of recounted, ill-received instruction, but Dave said it was basically a rinse and repeat of the first time. I'm not sure if he was just trying to make me feel better or not, but he said I might have done the second tube with one fewer practice. I often replay these moments in my head with slight humiliation.

All that effort and brain power definitely made me deserving of another nap.

At 1:17 p.m. on Saturday, Day 3, Dave sent the midday update:

> Our girl just woke up from her morphine nap from [after] the chest tube removal. She had some mashed potatoes, a little bit of a cookie and she fell back asleep.

More sleeping, more feeling uncomfortable, a few more bites of food, more repetitive conversation.

At 4:54 p.m. on Saturday, Day 3, Dave sent out his last update of the day:

> Evening update—short one here. All is well. Usual bit of uncomfortableness but everything is thumbs up.

He hung around with me for a few more hours and scooted out around 7 p.m. He called my mom on the way home, got settled in with the kitties and had another successful night's sleep.

Sunday morning, Day 4, Dave arrived with monster-sized cookies for the staff. He was the hero of the ICU!

At 10:50 a.m. on Sunday, Day 4, Dave sent his morning update:

> Sunday morning update—all the chest tubes are out and the central line is coming out later so she will be more mobile and can start walking around.

To the readers: how much faith do you have in me that I was able to understand and flawlessly execute the instructions for pulling out my last chest tube? My bet was on me doing it without any instruction at all. The sad reality is that I would have lost that bet. Dave says I wasn't quite as "stupid" as the first two times, but he still got a chuckle out of my persistent asking to practice before the real deal.

My PICC or "central" line came out shortly after the third and final chest tube. What is a PICC line? PICC stands for peripherally inserted central catheter. The thin tube (much larger than an IV line) was inserted into my jugular vein on the right side of my neck. The line was fed through my vein until it found its home near my heart. They use this line to administer medications. My arm veins were pretty congested with lines already, so this was the next best place to get the really good drugs close to my new, very sensitive, rejection-fighting heart.

Once we started weaning me off some of the medications, they were able to remove the PICC, the largest of my lines. There were no instructions for me to follow for this procedure. They knocked me right out. I was properly gowned up as if going into surgery again, my neck was cleaned and numbed, Dave was asked to leave, and they sedated me. When he came back in, by neck was bandaged up and I was one step closer to getting to roam the hospital halls–accompanied, of course.

Once I woke up from my PICC removal nap, I was finally pretty alert. I would still sleep on and off, but I was awake a lot more frequently. I was still asking the same five questions, and I was still often uncomfortable, but I was starting to feel like myself again, although myself with some new parts. Wow! It was still sinking in.

I would take short journeys in my brain. I would start with the realization that I have a healthy new heart, not the ultra-enlarged, malfunctioning, super inefficient old thing I was all too ready to get rid of. I would drift over to all the things I would be able to do again. Was running in the picture? Would I ever be able to finish that triathlon that eluded me 20+ years ago?

I would then slip into absolute gratitude for the donor and his or her family. The gift they gave me was well beyond anything I could truly comprehend. There is no textbook for how to feel when receiving someone else's heart. And then the empathy and sadness would trigger a small pool in my lower eyelids–realizing my donor family's grief and pain. They lost a son, or sister, or mom, or uncle.

Then a nurse would walk back in my room to take blood or give me pills (I was now able to take some orally), and I would snap back to the moment. I was pretty alert by the end of Day 4. I was still sleeping quite a bit, and I was definitely still struggling to lie comfortably, but every day was better than the one before. And in those first few days, in hindsight as I write this, I'm pretty stunned how quickly I bounced back. Just over two days post-surgery, all my tubes were out, and I was down to just IVs in both arms.

It was time for my first official walk. The physical therapist came in and showed me how to get out of bed on my own. This required leg muscles and my trusty, heart-shaped pillow. I was given very strict instructions NOT to use my arms to prop myself up. My ribcage was wired together, and muscles were still repairing themselves. If I used my arms, that could put pressure on my chest and potentially pop the wires or damage my chest. The thought of them potentially having to open me up to make repairs was all the incentive I needed to follow every instruction.

I grasped my pillow and held it close to my chest. I bent at the waist and pulled all my weight on my legs — mostly my thighs. I rocked myself forward and stood up without using my arms. It was a little ugly, but it got me upright.

They handed me a walker. I literally waved my hand as if shooing it out of my sight. I caught myself, remembered my manners, and said, "No thank you. I'd like to try without the walker." We took a lap around the ICU floor. My legs were pretty shaky, but I was doing it. I was walking! On my own, for a decent distance, and at a respectable pace.

At one point, the PT actually told me to slow down. I have never been a slow walker and it just didn't feel right to not be pushing my pace. I do remember being quite winded. The PT and I were talking as we were taking our lap, and I was getting a little out of breath. At about the halfway mark, I felt out of sorts, like too many things were happening at once. I was taking steps, forming sentences, breathing while talking, looking at and waving hello to the nurses. It was a lot of stimuli for one event.

We had a good round. I made it back to my room. And I didn't even lie to him when he asked me how I felt. I didn't do my usual. "I feel great. That was awesome! Piece of cake." Because frankly, it wasn't.

I admitted I was a bit winded and said the effort was a seven out of 10. I wanted it to be easy. I wanted it to be a one out of 10, but I knew this was all going to take time. No sense in trying to be super-woman. It was only day four, for goodness sakes. I could cut myself some slack.

As much as I wanted to lie back in bed, the occupational thera-pist was waiting and motioned me over to the sink in my room. She suggested I brush my teeth. I'd like to assume that it wasn't because I had raunchy breath, but because it was her job to help me improve my regular, everyday activities. Brushing my teeth was definitely a piece of cake. Her job was done!

Dave stayed a couple more hours, headed out around 7 p.m., and faithfully called my mom on the way home.

Monday morning, Dave showed up with a mix of muffins and cookies. It was seriously starting to make me jealous that the nurses were liking him more than me. OK, not really, but it was fun to say that in front of the staff. I loved seeing him so into the whole experi-ence. And it's never a bad thing to have your visitor be well-liked by the nurses. He was never reprimanded for staying a little late on those nights when we just weren't ready for him to leave.

At 11:36 on Monday, Day 5, Dave sent this:

> So upon my arrival, they were prepping her to go down for her chest x-ray. She was all smiles and feeling really good.

By this point, I was very alert, staying awake for long periods of time, learning how to position myself to be comfortable for more than 10 minutes at a time, and going to the bathroom unassisted. I finally brushed my hair for the first time in five days. It was a greasy, rats' nest mess and took at least 10 minutes to work the knots and matts out with a wide-tooth hair pick. It looked better but was no less greasy, and I think I was still several days from a shower. Sponge baths from the nurses would have to do for a while.

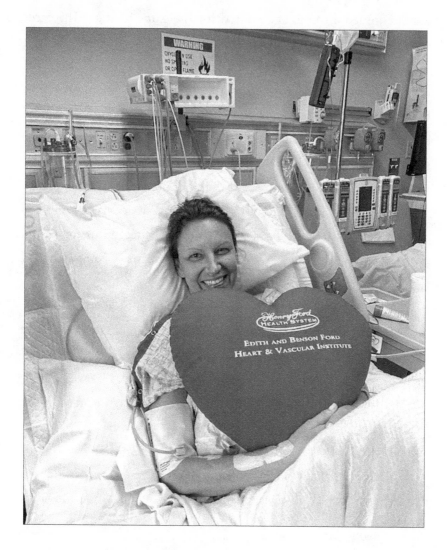

Now that I was awake more and with little to do, I grabbed my iPad and played a game of cards. I always love playing Spades, Hearts, and Euchre with live opponents. My mind was craving some mental stimulus, and my competitive, card-playing spirit was feeling a bit deprived. I flipped open the cover, hit the "on" button, clicked on Spades, joined a room, and waited for the game to start. The cards were delt, and it was my turn to bid my hand.

Bidding normally takes me about five seconds while I count the number of high face cards and spades, then type in my number. Oh boy! Not this time! My brain was mush. I couldn't focus. I recounted cards and spades several times. I was seeing messages fly across the screen, "Let's go!" and, "Hey, it's your turn." I placed my bid, but felt totally unsure that I accounted for the right number of cards. I played a couple hands (my less-than-patient opponent messaging me on-screen to hurry up) and closed the flap on my iPad. I'm sure my digital partner was irritated, but I was clearly not as mentally competent as I thought going into this.

A few minutes later, I opened my iPad and clicked on my Kindle app. Reading a book would be much less stressful. No one to irritate with my slow reaction time and no nasty responses to my poor judgment of which card to throw. I began reading a book that was recommended to me by several people. I was excited to get started. After reading the same six paragraphs at least four times, I gave up. Time to turn on the TV!

Dave and I talked. I asked more questions. My repertoire was expanding a bit. We ate dinner, and at 5:50 p.m. on Monday, Day 5, Dave sent this:

Evening update – all is good!!!! She had a good walk and stood for her x-ray.

Dave kissed me goodnight, walked to the garage, got into his car, called my mom on his way home, and had a restful night.

Chapter 9 – The Reunion

AT 8:47 AM ON Tuesday morning, Day 6, Dave wrote:

> Change up today. I am picking Kristy's mom up at the airport and taking her to the hospital so no morning update. Although I did talk to her for a moment, and she sounded great.

So why, you may ask, did it take my mom until day five to come see me? It was very important to her to be fully vaccinated for COVID-19 before she flew north. Fully vaccinated in March 2021 meant two shots. There was no booster yet. My mom lives in Florida. COVID vaccine appointments for her age category, which is a large part of Florida's population, were exceptionally difficult to schedule. She literally had eight of her friends who had created a COVID phone bank trying to make appointments for her and others.

She had a reaction to her first vaccine and wanted to be sure before she got on a plane to see me after her second shot that she wasn't experiencing symptoms while flying. That could make for a miserable three-and-a-half hours. She got her shot on Sunday, rode out Monday to ensure no reaction, and she was on a plane first thing Tuesday morning.

She and Dave called me from the airport to give me her ETA. I was beyond excited to see her. It had been 475 days since our last in-person visit. Damn COVID! I had played the scene over and over in my head. I kept envisioning it from her perspective. How would she feel walking in the room seeing her daughter on IVs, with a fat lip, scarred, bandaged, bruised, greasy hair, wearing a well-worn hospital gown, monitors everywhere?

Moments later, she walked into my room. It was magical! She did so great. No tears, just HUGE smiles from both of us. I reached my arms out toward her and as soon as she approached my bedside, we hugged. It was gentle — she knew better than to squeeze too tight — and we embraced for a good, long, satisfying, warm and fuzzy, forever memorable couple dozen seconds. It was so special!

As she was putting her things down and taking in the room, she was rattling off all the people who had sent me well wishes and was pulling things out of her bag. A friend gave her *this* to give me, and another friend gave her *that* to give me. She continued to root through her bag and pulled out something red and silky. She brought me a Superman cape! She had visions of me wearing it in the hospital. I felt slightly embarrassed to think she was going to "be a mom" and make me put it on in public. But I smiled sweetly, thanked her profusely and asked her to set it on the chair for the time being.

Within moments of her arrival, the PT and OT came to the room for my new daily routines. The PT said it was time for my walk, and I got to show off for my mom how well I could get out of the bed by myself. Out of the corner of my eye I saw her cringe a bit in an empathetic attempt to feel any discomfort I may be feeling. And as any mama bear would, she lurched forward in an attempt to help me when I grimaced at the point when my thigh muscles had to engage, *sans assistance* from my hands, to get upright. She restrained herself and let me do it on my own.

As I took my first few steps and was about to disappear with the PT, she said, "Wait! Your cape! You have to wear this on your walk." I'm so glad she was busy reaching for it when I did a classic eye roll! But when she turned around with the cape in hand, I was smiling at her. She so proudly placed the cape on my back, tied it at my neck and hugged me gently. I began to walk and she again said, "Wait!" I stopped, she grabbed her phone, and snapped a picture. I guarantee she has looked at that picture at least 50 times since that day. A #proudmama moment for sure!

She posted this picture on Facebook and made sure to point out that I was walking faster than the PT. Can you see where I got my competitive spirit?!

I was a little less out of breath on this round. I also climbed several stairs. Because I was holding my IV pole, I could only go up and down about four steps, but I did it several times. I was a little out of breath, but I felt pretty darn good. I walked back to the room, brushed my teeth under the supervision of my OT, washed my face, and got myself back into bed not nearly as exhausted as last time.

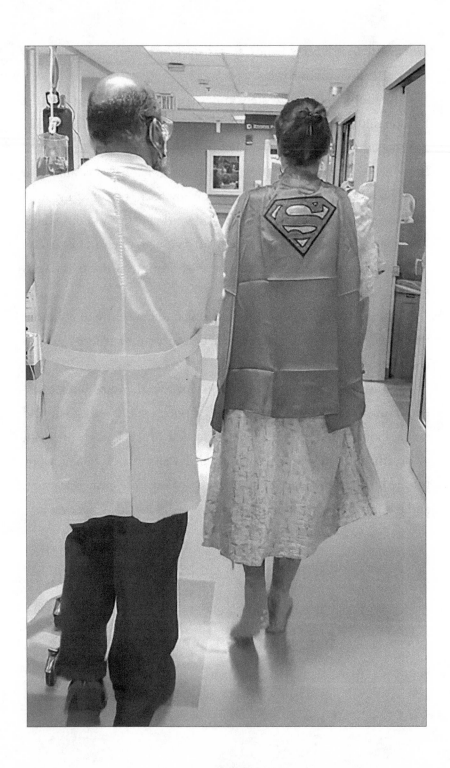

Within the hour of my walk, Dr. Nemeh came in. My mom was like a star-struck fan in his presence. There is no way to put into words the extent of gratitude a mom would have for a man who saved her daughter's life and gave her a second chance. She was composed and gracious and lovely with him, using the perfect words and phrases to thank him.

The reason for his visit on this particular day was to show me the x-ray comparisons. He pulled up his phone, scrolled through his photo gallery, and excitedly and proudly handed me his phone. With a huge smile, he said:

"Look at your beautiful new heart. And look at your old heart." He looked at my face and waited for it to register.

Holy shit! I had been told for years how enlarged my heart was. Several doctors had told me how stunned they were to see it. It was huge! (I always like to think when they said I had a huge heart that they were referring to how kind I was.) Stories were recounted from other doctors how my heart may have been the largest they had ever seen, especially for someone as seemingly heathy as I was. Nothing could have prepared me for what I saw in these side-by-side x-ray photos.

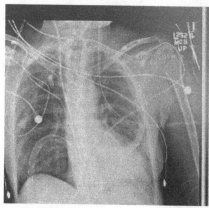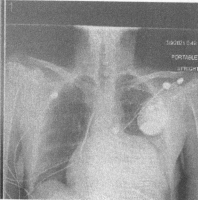

Look at the photo on the right. My heart was taking up almost half of my entire thorax. It was spilling over into the right side of my chest cavity. It was enormous. Compare it to the x-ray on the left. My new heart looks so dainty. I have actually had people look at these pictures and ask where my heart even is in that picture. You can barely see it. I still can't believe the difference when I look at these pictures.

You may also notice in the picture on the right that there is a small white blob above my huge blob of a heart. That was my defibrillator. Notice it is gone now. It took me months to get used to the concept of not having it anymore. That device was part of me for more than 20 years. At first, realizing I didn't have it was a little alarming. It was always my safety net. I no longer need it. That seemed extremely strange. It was awesome, but hard to get used to.

You know the other thing that was really hard for me to get used to? Saying I *had* heart disease. Or saying I *had* ARVC. I don't have heart disease anymore! And it took me months to get used to talking about my cardiac issues as being in the past. Weird, but wonderful!

As Mom and I were getting settled, the sweetest thing happened. A delivery arrived for me. The ICU doesn't allow for patients to receive live flowers, yet a nurse was walking toward me with a gorgeous bouquet. My wonderful colleagues sent me a gift from a company called Unwilted. I would strongly encourage you to check them out. They make beautiful, everlasting paper flower arrangements. This gift brightened my room instantly.

Mom and I savored our time together for the rest of the afternoon. We talked about the latest with our family members and her friends, I napped, we had lunch, I napped, we caught up on her life over the last six days, I napped, we laughed, we had dinner, then Dave came to pick her up and take her home. This was Day One of their (our) 70 days together.

It is hospital policy that a transplant patient has two caretakers for 90 days. That meant my husband living with his mother-in-law for three months. I am so grateful they get along, truly love each other, and are both patient people. It doesn't matter how much you like someone; it takes serious patience and respect to live with a person other than your spouse for weeks on end. And for my mom who is an extremely social and active person to leave her friends, her significant other, and all the activities she loves in Florida to weather a winter in Michigan was a huge sacrifice, I know.

After Mom left, I had my worst night yet. I was far from tired, I was extremely restless and uncomfortable, and I could not get myself to feel settled for the night. I watched two movies (the first time I had turned on my TV in almost a week). After *Pitch Perfect 3* and *Rocketman*, it was now after midnight. I couldn't believe I still wasn't ready to go to sleep.

During the movies, I had called the nurse a few times to arrange my pillows. My restlessness once again would cause things to shift, so I was ready to call for the nurse again. I went to grab my call button and when I moved my arm toward the device, I knocked it on the floor. "*Dammit!*" I couldn't reach it. I tried to hang onto the bed rail and scoot myself off the side of the bed to reach it. I thought I was close, tried to reach a bit farther and gave up when I remembered how the PT had told me that reaching too far before my chest healed could cause my wires to be displaced. The thought made me shudder. I maneuvered back to a lying position and did the only thing I could do — moan/whine for the nurse.

"Nurse!"

Nothing.

"Hello!"

No one.

"Help, please."

Silence.

"Can someone please help me?"

Zero movement in the hall.

Frustration. Patience. Close my eyes and chill. Wait. Regain some sense of calm.

Finally, the nurse came in. I told her I needed help getting comfortable. She handed me the call button. I wrapped the cord around my bedrail so it couldn't fall again. She did an amazing job with my pillows. I thanked her. I closed my eyes. I willed myself to go to sleep. Nothing. That is when my HGTV marathon started. Five episodes in a row. Ugh. It was 2:45 a.m. I turned the TV off and finally fell asleep shortly after that.

"How are your sleep patterns?" the PT asked the next day, Wednesday, Day 7. Did I look particularly haggard that morning?

"Honestly, they're pretty lousy," I told him. I told him about my really rough night. He gave me some great advice.

"Get yourself in a position of not sleeping as much during the day," he said, "and try to sleep at night. You need to get back to a normal rhythm."

Dave showed up shortly after that, with cookies and muffins, of course. He kissed me and said he wanted to show me something. He took out his phone and opened up his photo gallery. He handed it to me, and my eyes welled up with tears.

Two of my friends had snuck over to our house the day before and filled the front lawn with signs. They sporadically and abundantly scattered red hearts all over the yard, planted a sign that said "Kristy Strong," and another one that said "You Go, Girl!" My favorite was three huge emojis:

I was overwhelmed by the thought that these two took time out of their busy lives to: A) create such thoughtful signs; and B) go to my house in 30-degree weather to post them all over my front yard.

Then Dave asked how I slept. I recounted my awful night and told him what the PT said. Dave was a great partner, keeping me awake and occupied all day. I slept for about 45 minutes during a dumb movie we watched together, but other than that, I stayed awake the entire day. That was a great turning point for getting my sleeping patterns back on track.

On Wednesday during rounds, the on-call doc and her entourage of residents came in for the usual show. Just like you see on TV. She would read my chart, share the highlights with the residents, one of them would speak up and ask me questions, she would fire off a few questions to the rest of the group, she would do a quick exam, share with me her assessment, and end by asking if I had any questions. This day I got bold and asked, "When can I go home?" She gave me the best news ever:

"Most patients' recovery is 10 to 14 days," she said, "but I'm feeling pretty good that you'll be out in a couple more days. I'll shoot for Friday."

I was elated. Dave and I were grinning at each other like a couple school kids.

Before she scooted out, she said she wanted to show us some pictures. Dave got all excited. I was a little non-plussed, because I assumed they were the same x-rays Dr. Nemeh showed me yesterday.

"I have pictures of your new heart and your old heart," she said.

Dave bounded up off the edge of my bed. He couldn't wait to see them. She brought the phone over to both of us. I caught a half-second glimpse before snapping my head away in disbelief. She was showing us actual photos of my old heart. I had ZERO interest. And to this day I still have not looked at them. Dave describes it like this:

They were all "live" photos where the first couple seconds show actual movement. The first picture she showed him was of my old heart. It was on a stainless steel OR table covered with a surgical cloth. It was shocking in the fact that it just didn't look like a heart. It was a large yellowish, fatty blob that was still slightly beating. He said it was indistinguishable — didn't even look like an organ. My ventricle was huge and it clearly looked unhealthy.

The next picture was my new heart on a tray with surgical cloth underneath it. In the few seconds of live motion, Dave could see the doctors tying something to it. It was red, pink, and white. He could distinguish the chambers and one of the primary arteries; it looked like a normal, healthy, right-sized heart. (Thank goodness!)

The last picture, although out of order, was of my old heart in my chest... beating. Gross! I am so glad I did not see any of this. Dave was fascinated. He asked Dr. Jennifer Cowger if she could send them to him. I think Dave became her medical nerd pal at that point. She was so happy that at least one of us was interested in her team's miraculous handiwork. An hour later they showed up in Dave's inbox. He shows them to anyone who will indulge him. I am still not one of them.

Dave and I had a normal day. I finally started making some phone calls. My first call was to my high school best friend. It was an emotional call. I was acutely aware of how my voice sounded. It was very shaky. I blamed it on the sentimentality of the conversation. But even after we got past the mushy stuff and we were laughing and talking about non-transplant, catch-up topics, I kept thinking that I sounded like Katherine Hepburn. I asked Dave after I hung up if he had noticed it. He said he had. I chalked it up to just being weak, but it was really annoying me.

After a really good day, Dave headed home. No call to my mom this time, since he would see her at the house in less than 30 minutes. The next day, Day 8, Thursday, was her day to be with me.

Chapter 10 – The Countdown

THURSDAY MORNING STARTED REALLY early! It was time for my very first of what would ultimately be at least 15 to 20 heart biopsies. The purpose of a biopsy is to determine, through tissue samples, if my body is rejecting my heart. They came to get me around 6:30 a.m. They wheeled me for what seemed like 10 minutes down hallways, on an elevator, through secure doorways, into the heart cath department. They prepped me by hooking me up to an EKG, a blood pressure monitor, and a pulse oximeter on my finger. Then they ran through all my meds and explained the procedure. Next, I waited until it was my turn to be wheeled in.

I had had a number of heart caths before. These were all done to scope out the inside of my heart. In the past, they had always gone through a vein in my groin or my arm. Today (and every time since) they would go in through the jugular vein in my neck. At 7:30, they wheeled me back to the freezing cold lab. It looked like all other cath labs I'd been in–it was basically a mini OR.

A team behind the glass was recording everything and the team that would be performing the procedure and assisting the doc were on the main floor with me. The toughest part of the whole procedure was having to move myself from the hospital bed onto the cath table. Remember, I had no use of my arms, and was not able to roll completely on my side for fear of crushing my chest, or widening my chest too much. *Ay yay yay.*

The staff helped me, but it was pretty ugly. I was now on the table.

"Move your body closer to the top," they said. "Get more in the center, and lift your head so we can straighten the pillow."

Finally, all was right with the positioning of my body.

The crew was super energetic and fun. We were yuckin' it up. I got to pick the playlist; I asked for 90's alternative. They adjusted my EKG leads and put the defibrillator pads on me (precaution in case something with my heart rhythm went awry). They were adjusting monitors and getting the instruments ready. They did their formal time-out: this is when they stated my name, recited my medical record number, indicated the time, explained the procedure, announced which doctor was performing the biopsy, and had everyone verbally agree.

They started my sedation, which honestly had virtually no effect on me–it never did for these procedures. I was fully alert. The doc came in, introduced himself, got in position on the right side of my neck, and announced, "Little prick and a burn. I'm numbing the area where we're inserting the catheter." I felt the prick, didn't really feel the burn, and heard them doing their thing.

They inserted a sheath into my vein, slid the catheter into the opening of the sheath, and fed the catheter through my vein into my heart. The first half of the procedure involved a right heart analysis. They scoped around and announced a bunch of numbers and readings that meant nothing to me. The right heart cath took all of 10 minutes. They pulled the catheter out and attached a little set of pinchers on the end. I was not able to see what they were doing, but I have since asked them to show me pretty much every component of the procedure. With each biopsy, I would get more curious. For this first one, I just laid still and let them do their things. We were chatting and laughing during the procedure. If I remember right, the theme of this first biopsy was music.

So back to the procedure. The little "scissors" were now on the end of the catheter. They fed it back through the sheath and back into my vein, down to my right ventricle. They placed the pinchers on the wall of my ventricle and snipped a tiny piece of tissue. I didn't feel anything that resembled pain or cutting, but my heart fluttered a bit. I now know that the heart didn't appreciate the doc coming in and stealing part of it, so it decided to throw off a couple irregular beats. It was a bit uncomfortable for me, but I've lived with irregular beats for more than two decades now. No big deal. They pulled the catheter out, placed the tissue sample into a small vial, and headed back in for sample number two. For this biopsy, they took three samples. The whole procedure took less than a half hour.

The doc announced, "OK. We're all done. We'll have your results in a couple days." He left and the staff removed everything they hooked me up to.

"You can scootch back on to the bed," they said. They wheeled me back to the main area where the nurse pulled the sheath out of my vein, held pressure on it for 10 minutes, and bandaged up the little hole in my neck. They wheeled me back up to my room.

What were they looking for during a biopsy? They were able to tell from the donor DNA whether or not my body was rejecting the heart. If I showed signs of rejection, they would adjust my meds. The first time I heard the term "rejection" in relation to my own new heart, I was terrified. I thought that meant they would have to open me back up and give me a new heart. Heart transplant patients have an average of one to three rejection episodes within the first year, and

50% to 80% of transplant recipients experience at least one rejection episode. It's not as dire as it sounds. They perform biopsies so they can stay ahead of any problems and make adjustments quickly.

Back in my room, I took a little nap and was awakened by my mom tiptoeing toward me. I looked up. She smiled and put her hand on my forehead. Shortly after she arrived, Dr. Cowger was back again with her gaggle of residents and some really great news: "Looks like you should be able to go home tomorrow, but if not tomorrow, since that will be Friday, we'll have to wait until Monday."

As I'm sure you can imagine, I had zero interest in waiting until Monday. If I were given the sliver of hope that I could be going home on Friday, eight days after my surgery, I was going to do everything possible to make that happen. Part of me just wanted to be home. Part of me wanted out of the hospital. The competitive part of me wanted to be discharged in record time. So few patients get out before 10 days post-transplant. I could do it in eight! Monday would mean 11. No way. That just wouldn't do.

Be an A patient, Kristy! Get sprung early!

The penultimate step before leaving the hospital was to be moved from my current ICU to what they called a step-down room. It was still part of the ICU floor, but it didn't have all the monitoring equipment and hookups like the ICU room I had spent the last week in. It was the dream move. Successfully spend a day in step-down, and you were free to go home. The finish line was feeling so close.

While they were making arrangements to move me, it was time to meet with the nutritionist and the pharmacist. Let me just say how absolutely grateful I was that my mom was there to endure these over-stimulating, information-overload sessions with me. My mom worked in the medical and rehab profession for many years and was such a valuable ear as we were flooded with information. My mom, being very inquisitive, is a practiced clarifier and an excellent note-taker. I was not in the state of mind to be any of these things.

The pharmacist came first. I would leave the hospital taking 32 pills a day. Tell me that didn't require some brain power to absorb! Here I was, still in a little post-transplant fog, having to comprehend all of these medicines that were now about to be part of my everyday life. I needed to understand what they were called, what they were for, when I was supposed to take them, what side effects I might get, whether I was supposed to take them with food or not.

I learned which ones could upset my stomach, cause diabetes or high blood pressure, or raise my cholesterol, which one could give me tremors. Tremors, and a shaky voice! *Yep – already got that one!*

The vast amount of information coming at me was daunting. Thankfully, I was taking notes. My mom was taking notes. Hers were much more legible. We had a binder of information to take with us, which was helpful, but after an hour with the pharmacist, my head felt like I needed a brain transplant!

Next was the nutritionist. I pride myself on being a very healthy eater, so I thought round two would be a piece of cake. No way would this session require much thought or concentration. WRONG! There are so many things I am now restricted from eating.

No grapefruit, pomegranate, or blood orange because they have interactions with my drugs.

Nothing raw, so no sushi, which really bummed me out. I could at least have cooked sushi–even smoked salmon. That was a bit of sil-ver lining! No lunch meat. All meats had to be fully cooked and at the proper temperature when I consume them. I had to eat all beef well done. Seriously?! I love me a good medium rare steak or burger (the infrequent times I actually eat them). Undercooked meats have the potential of having bacteria that could get into my now very delicate, ill-equipped, immune-compromised system. My immune system had become so suppressed, if I got sick, it would be very difficult to fight it off.

All fruits and vegetables had to be thoroughly washed. Dave had been on my case our entire married life about how I rarely wash my fruits and vegetables. I'd always had an exceptionally strong immune system and actually preferred to know that I was eating a little bit of dirt and bacteria because I just felt it kept my immune system strong. I hardly ever was sick pre-transplant. Dave and my mom had really started to get on my case about washing my produce, probably about a year pre-transplant. So, I had started to get into the habit, but man, did this nutritionist put the fear of God and me about not eating anything that wasn't thoroughly washed. My mom felt vindicated, I'm sure! Other fruits and vegetables that were totally off limits were cantaloupe and sprouts. Too much potential for dirt to get trapped in crevices that couldn't be reached or properly cleaned.

The more I thought about the seriousness of not consuming bacteria, the more bummed I got when thinking about eating out. I love to eat salads at restaurants, but they told me, "Unless you know they're really thoroughly washing the vegetables, you're going to have to pass on eating fresh produce outside of your own kitchen."

I was told I couldn't eat anything past the expiration date (another thing I was famous for taking risks with). I couldn't eat anything unpasteurized and now needed to be sure that all cheeses (and I love interesting cheeses) were safe for me. No licking the cookie dough bowl–no raw eggs for me. Again–bacteria.

I was also reminded of some of the things shared with me by the infectious disease doc during my pre-transplant work-up: no gardening (I could breathe in bacteria in the dirt); no changing the cat litter (hooray); no changing bird feeders, because of the bacteria in bird poop (bummer, since I'm a total bird nerd).

That was a helluva back-to-back two hours of brain-numbing information intake. Even my mom looked like she had more than she could take. She felt a very strong sense of responsibility to take all this information and be my teacher, supervisor, and counselor over the next few months as I tried to break old habits and remember all of these new routines.

Mom went down and bought some lunch for us and by the time she returned, we got the green light to move to my new room. Between my mom and the nurse, we grabbed all my things and headed to my new, hopefully one-day-only, step-down digs. They wheeled my bed, with me in it, across the ICU floor. They pushed me through the threshold and Mom and I looked at each other as if I'd just been shown to the presidential suite at the Grand Hotel in Mackinac Island, Michigan. OK, it wasn't really "grand" but it was huge, and bright, and lacking all the machines and equipment and dependence-inducing devices I had gotten so used to in my other room.

We ate, and the pharmacist came back for round two. *Ugh. There's more?* As much as I was disappointed that we weren't done, it was honestly great to have another walk-through. She had the actual medicine bottles with her, and she showed me my new lifeline–the weekly pill case with seven individual pop-out containers, each with four compartments that corresponded to the four times a day I would be taking my drugs: 7 a.m., 9 a.m., 9 p.m., and 10 p.m. It was a very worthwhile session.

Just about as soon as she left, the OT came by for our daily session. She looked at me, smiled slyly and said, "I'm not really sure what we're going to do today. You've passed all the milestones. You're brushing your teeth, you're combing your hair. You can manage yourself in the bathroom. You kind of do it all now! Is there anything you can think of you want to do?"

I excitedly responded with, "You know what I would really love right now? I would love it if I could take a shower, shave my legs, and wash my hair."

"I can't let you take a shower," she said, "but I'd be happy to wash your hair."

I happily agreed to her compromise. She moved a chair into the shower room and I took a seat. I was wearing my hospital gown, and she wrapped a towel around my shoulders between my body and the back of the chair. I leaned my head back and enjoyed the most satisfying shampooing of my life. This, after nine days of not being able to wash my hair and keeping it up in a bun, it was feeling pretty disgusting.

My mom was waiting in the main room, and all of a sudden she gasped, "Oh my gosh! Guys! The room is flooding!"

The OT explained that when they built this whole wing of rooms, they didn't take into account any grading of the floor, so my room was flooding all the way out into the ICU hallway. My mom started gathering all the towels she could find; the OT went into the hall and grabbed some blankets. Between the two of them, they sopped up an 18-foot stream of water. They detained the flood from seeping past the threshold and to the rest of the hospital.

All this was happening around me, and all I could think of was how amazing it felt to have a squeaky clean head of hair, now conditioned, silky smooth, and primed for a comb to glide right through.

After profusely thanking the OT, and her wishing me well, she headed off to see her next patient. Mom and I spent a bit more time together, then she was ready to head home so she could eat a proper dinner with Dave. We were both so excited about the prospect that the next time we would see each other would be at the house tomorrow.

She remained with me while I ate dinner off the hospital menu. I don't remember what it was, but I can assure you it was awful. My nurse came in shortly after my food was delivered. He was really cool, and we had been joking around much of the afternoon. I decided to ask him if he had ever eaten their hospital food. He confidently and proudly said, "Never!"

I responded with, "Well, today is your lucky day!" With every meal I was given this small plastic container of protein gelatin. The first time they served it, I decided to try it. Jell-O can be edible, and a little protein seemed like a bonus. I could not have been more wrong! Oh my God, I gagged when I first tried it. And never again did I even attempt to remove the foil from the plastic cup that housed this almost neon-colored, firm-yet-jiggly concoction.

So now, I took the familiar plastic container off my tray and handed it to my nurse. He looked at me. He looked at my mom. He smiled and made sure I knew I was the only patient he had ever done this for. He peeled the foil off, and I handed him my unused spoon. My mom and I smiled at each other (because yes, I had made her try it too a couple days earlier). He put a small portion into his mouth, chewed (if that's what you actually do with Jell-O), and started making a face before he even swallowed. His grimace lingered for a couple more seconds until we all busted out laughing. I coyly apologized.

My mom headed home shortly after dinner, then the PT came in for our last session. He showed me warm-up and cool-down exercises. This had been explained before, but it didn't really sink in. A transplanted heart works differently than a "normal" heart. When my old heart was removed, the vagal nerve was severed. In most heart transplant patients, those nerves don't regenerate.

They attached my new heart to a denervated nerve. This means that unlike you, when you start to exercise or exert yourself, your vagal nerve immediately indicates to your heart that it needs to start pumping faster. With a transplanted heart, my nerve doesn't function anymore, so it can't tell the heart to beat faster. I have to wait for my body to produce adrenaline that will eventually travel to my brain and instruct it to tell my heart to beat faster.

This means that any time I'm going to exercise, I have to warm up first. He showed me a routine of four pre- and post-walk exercises: arm raises, knee raises, toe raises, and rocking back and forth between the balls of my feet and my heels.

He explained how he wanted me to increase my activity over the next few months.

"When you get home tomorrow," he said, "you should walk for seven minutes at least twice a day. You can increase by two minutes every day. You can walk more than twice if you want to. You should always warm up and cool down with the series I just taught you."

"Can I walk outside?" I asked.

"Not until you can walk for 20 minutes straight," he said. "I don't want you in a situation where you get too far away from the house and are not able to walk back. I also don't want you on uneven surfaces."

I asked what I thought was the next logical question, "So I just walk on my treadmill?"

He shot back a very firm, "No!" Until I was able to walk at cardiac rehab, monitored, I was not allowed to get on my treadmill.

My brain was calculating what he was saying. Bottom line, and he validated this when I said it a bit in disbelief, "So you're saying I have to walk around the inside of my house for up to 20 minutes, two to three times a day, before I can go outside? Can I at least go up and down stairs to get some variety around the house?"

"No! Other than going up to your bedroom at the end of the day, I don't want you climbing stairs. You need to walk around your main floor."

Oh, boy! Can you say B-O-R-I-N-G?

He watched me perform my new warm-up series, then we went for a couple laps around the ICU floor. After observing my cool down, he wished me well as he left for the last time. I felt good, I felt eager, I felt motivated, and I felt like everything was sinking in.

I'm going home tomorrow and am about to start a really long, really slow, underwhelmingly-paced recovery, but a recovery nonetheless. I was so grateful for what was ahead. Grateful! Thoughts of my donor family seeped in again. I put my hands over the left side of my chest, closed my eyes, and let thoughts of gratitude for my donor and his/her family fill my mind. This has since become a daily ritual for me.

I settled into bed, a little more able to find a comfortable position for sleeping. I attempted a couple games on my iPad, not playing against live opponents this time. I learned that lesson! I called Dave and asked him to pack a few things for me to wear home tomorrow. I was so close. And I was so hopeful that tomorrow would play out the way we all wanted so I could go home.

Before I shut off my light for the night, I posted to The Transplant Tribune, the Facebook group I created before my surgery but hadn't touched since. Dave had been the master updater on this medium as well. It was kind of exciting to take it back over, and what I wrote was such an incredible walk down memory lane. And in case you want the *Cliff Notes* version of the last couple chapters, here's what I wrote:

OK. It's looking to be true. I'm planning to leave the hospital tomorrow!!

Timeline:

- Weekend of March 6 and 7 — sustained irregular rhythms

- Mon, March 8 — day in ER to stabilize me then transferred to Henry Ford

- Tues, March 9 — officially on the transplant list

- Wed, March 10 — found a heart

- Thurs, March 11 — transplant

- Thurs, Sat, March 11-13 — various tube removal (this part is pretty foggy for me)

- Sun-Wed, March 14-17 — PT, OT, lots of meds, my first biopsy for anti-rejection results

- Today, Thurs — education overload! Nutrition, pharma, self-care, side effects, timelines, what to avoid, lifestyle changes, etc., and the best hair wash ever!!!

Tomorrow my final lines and IVs will be removed, and I will be chauffeured home in the back seat with my big fluffy chest pillow between my bod and the seatbelt.

Then the doc appointments, lab work, cardiac rehab, med adjustments, and extra precautions go into overdrive while my new chapter begins. I feel like the last week has been a cakewalk compared to what is ahead of me. I recognize virtually nothing about my body right now

- the bruises, the scars, the swelling, the atrophy, and this beautiful new heart inside of me. I can't wait to get to know it intimately and push it in ALL THE RIGHT ways.

I appreciate my support network more than ever. Thank you, all, sooooooo much! I am forever grateful to you for staying by my side through this first critical phase. Stay tuned...

Friday morning started with one final milestone before Dave arrived. The last thing that needed to be done before they let me go was to remove the pacemaker wire from my chest. Why did I need a pacemaker? They had just gotten rid of my defibrillator/pacemaker during my transplant. The practice of inserting a temporary pacemaker was common immediately post-transplant. The heart was still learning to beat effectively on its own and it needed a little assistance while all my new parts were beginning to work together harmoniously. It was one more safety net in the early days.

What I found fascinating, and a bit disturbing, was that they wanted to keep my heart beating at a steady 110 beats per minute right after transplant. And even after removing the wire, it would always beat around 100 bpm. The nerves leading to my heart had been cut, and this caused a more rapid heart rate... from here on out. My exercise heart rate would also take a lot longer to elevate, just like the PT told me the night before.

Why was this such a big adjustment for me? Prior to my transplant and for most of my 20 years living with ARVC, my resting heart rate was between 45 and 50 beats per minute. Part of the reason for the slow rate was because I was still relatively fit, but most of it was due to my medications that lowered my heart rate and BP.

So just imagine the sensation difference–I went from a slow, weak beat to a rate that was more than double what I had been used to for the last two decades. Not only was it faster, but it was robust and strong and forceful. It was something I was suddenly very conscious of. This time, however, being conscious of my heart rhythm was a positive thing. Since my first heart issues in my twenties, feeling my heart rhythm was always a negative thing. I had lived almost half my life being conscious of how my heart was beating. It was never positive. This was another beautiful reminder of the new me!

My nurse walked in. The same one from yesterday. His first comment, even before saying good morning, was, "Do you have any idea how long that awful taste lingered in my mouth yesterday? It was the first story I recounted to my wife when I got home."

It reminded me of a line I learned in my public relations class in college: *love me or hate me, but just don't ignore me.* He may not have loved me yesterday, but something tells me he won't ever forget me. I apologized, but I'm not going to lie... I did laugh!

"It's time to remove your pacemaker line," he said. I was very alert and admittedly a little anxious. They were pulling out a wire that had been happily living inside my heart for more than a week. My nurse prepped me with a sterilizing solution and told me to lie really still. It wasn't painful, but I absolutely felt the sensations within my heart and on the surface of my skin as he pulled the four-inch wire from my body.

He immediately put a bandage on it.

"Lay still for 30 minutes," he said. "I'll be back to check on you then. If everything is stable, that's the final indicator that you can leave the hospital and go home."

While I was lying still, Dave arrived — with muffins! He brought the few things I asked for the night before. My friend's brother who had recently had a heart transplant taught me a few very valuable lessons. One of them was that due to the fluids, and the drugs, and the inactivity, he was quite swollen when he left the hospital. I too had noticed my bloated belly among other unrecognizable traits. The form-fitting joggers I had on the day I was admitted to the ER (my God, that felt like forever ago) would not be comfortable, if I could even get them on. Dave brought me some super loose-fitting lounge pants. Fingers crossed I would actually be able to wear them in a few hours.

Assuming the best, Dave began packing up my things. Dr. Cowger came in and said I was good to go. They were typing up my discharge papers. This was really happening! I had a final consult with her while she told me for the fifth or sixth time all the things that I needed to do when I left the hospital. Two or three of them I honestly didn't remember from before, so repetition, although it made me feel a little inferior, was actually a good thing.

So, who, you may wonder, is this Dr. Cowger? And what happened to Dr. Lanfear? I had wondered the same thing a few days earlier. Dr. Lanfear was my great pre-transplant guy, then I spent my amazing day with my surgeons, and now I have a post-transplant doc. She would be my main medical professional from here on out.

Kristy 2.0 was leaving the building! As I was dressing in my baggy clothes and ridding myself of a hospital gown after almost two weeks, I took note of every inch of my body. This was very difficult for me. I saw multiple bruises, scars, swollen lower legs, a bloated belly, and atrophied muscles in my arms and upper legs. Plus, my feet were red (almost purple). Who was I? Much of what I saw resulted from my new medications. And I thought they told me my liver would go back to normal size right away. I guess "right away" was a relative term.

As unnerving as it was to see my body this way, I was really proud of myself when I pushed the negativity out of my brain and quickly shifted my thinking to:

This is temporary.

My body is like this for a reason. I didn't overeat or miss workouts. I have no control over what I look like right now.

This is not my body – it has been taken over by meds and fluids and incisions and insertions.

In fact, the reason I look like this is a beautiful thing. I am alive. I have a new heart. I have a new life!

This internal conversation was the beginning of the end of so much wasted energy focusing on the negative about my body for almost 35 years. In the grand scheme of things, it was so petty; it was useless and counterproductive. It was time to take this new "ugliness" and turn it into something positive. I wasn't going to turn off many old habits overnight, but I had this burning confidence that my mind was shifting in this very moment. More about this later.

Let's get the heck out of this hospital first.

I, of course, said my goodbyes to my doctors and my nurses. They had become my new medical family. One of my nurses called the porter, and Dave went down to get the car. He too made his round of the ICU floor and said goodbye and thanked everyone. The porter arrived five minutes later with my wheelchair.

As I was being wheeled to the elevator, I reflected on so many things about the last week-and-a-half since I was first brought in by ambulance. The overall experience at the hospital was incredible. The staff was amazing. Everyone — from the people who came to take out my trash, to the people who cheerfully brought me my horrific hospital food, to the techs who took my x-rays in my room or who wheeled me off for other tests. The people who came in at all hours to check my vitals, give me heparin shots in my stomach so I wouldn't form blood clots; the multiple nurses, assistants and phlebotomists who came in multiple times a day to draw my blood; and the staff who came in on very strict schedules to administer my drugs four times a day. It took an army to get me to this point, and truly everybody was incredible.

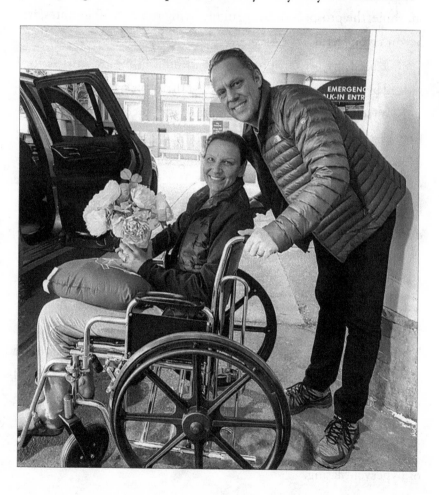

The porter and I chit-chatted on the long ride down to the valet area. He asked when I had my surgery, and I told him "a week ago yesterday." He was stunned. It was the beginning of the many times I would spark disbelief from people as they asked me to tell the stories of my transplant and recovery. The overachiever was alive and well and working every day to retain that status!

Dave pulled up in the car. He hopped out at the same time the porter wheeled me toward him. The fresh, cold air on my face, the sunshine, the prospect of being in my living room in 30 minutes, was beyond wonderful.

I used my get-out-of-the-chair-without-using-my-arms skills. I walked by myself to the car, Dave opened the door, and I slowly maneuvered myself into the backseat of the car. I was not allowed to sit in the front seat for six to eight weeks. The potential of an airbag going off and damaging the handiwork done by the surgeons was way too risky.

That's cool. I can be chauffeured. I placed my trusty red heart pillow between my chest and the seatbelt. Dave gave me a kiss, closed the door, and swiftly walked to the driver's seat.

He looked back at me, smiled sweetly, and said, "Let's get you home!" We pulled out of the hospital campus, entered the freeway, and started making our way toward our house, where my mom was patiently waiting for us.

About five minutes after we got onto the freeway, the magnitude of what had just happened hit me like a ton of bricks. My eyes welled up with tears, my throat felt tight, I rolled the window down trying to get extra air in my lungs (even though it was a mid-March winter day in Michigan). All of the sudden I was sobbing. I was on the verge of hyperventilating.

I'm not much of a crier in normal situations, but this was no normal situation. I could not control myself. Dave whipped his head around.

"Do I need to pull over?" he asked, as stunned at the onset of this as I was. I couldn't really speak, but somehow I indicated that he was OK to keep driving. The empathy on his face was beautifully and painfully welcomed.

The weight of what had just happened was suddenly and agonizingly all-consuming. Someone lost their life and gifted it to me. A family was grieving for someone they would never witness living again.

I am now living as a result of their grief.

I also began reflecting about how I had just endured one of the most intense medical procedures ever performed. I not only came through it, but I was thriving. The fact that I now had a whole new life ahead of me was so overwhelming. At that moment, I wasn't sure I was ever going to be able to stop crying. I had never felt like this before.

Dave looked back again. "Should I stop the car so I can come sit in the backseat with you?"

I was finally able to speak. Barely. "I'll be fine. I just need to process everything."

I cried for a good five minutes straight, whimpered for probably another five more, and pulled myself together — mostly. I had a sudden urge to document this moment for "the world." I pulled out my phone, pulled up the Transplant Tribune on Facebook, and created a post. It included a few pictures of me getting into the car... all smiles. The comments were flooding back at me fast and furious. One of my friends responded with "SURREAL!"

I responded with: "You have no idea. I am sitting in the back of the car bawling my eyes out. I will never be able to put this day into words."

I called my mom to warn her that I might be an emotional wreck when I walked into the house. I told her about my came-from-nowhere, totally-out-of-control breakdown and that seeing her could quite possibly trigger another one. Ten minutes later, we pulled into the driveway. I recognized the yard signs from my friends. Wait! These are totally new signs! These were welcome home signs, and there were red balloons and big red hearts staked all over the yard. I felt so loved!

Chapter 11 – The Homecoming

WE WALKED IN THE front door. I gently hugged my mom. No tears. No breakdown. Dave carried my things in, since I was not allowed to lift anything heavier than a gallon of milk. He too, hugged my mom while I made my way to the place where I was about to spend a huge percentage of my time over the next three or four months — our family room couch.

Once I got settled, my mom and Dave started a bit of show and tell. I was floored! In the last couple days, I had received flowers, care packages of soup and cookies, blankets, fuzzy slippers, lotions, coloring books, tea, mugs, candles, lip balm, and other super thoughtful goodies. I was overwhelmed by the love and support of my friends and family. I have since created a list of all the amazing companies and creative things people sent so I can pay it forward to others when they need their day brightened.

I hung with my family for a few hours, opening gifts, sending texts and emails to friends and family, letting everyone know I was home. The feeling of being in my own house with two of the people I love most in the world was the best homecoming I could have asked for. I lasted a few more hours and decided it was time to call it quits for the day.

The last thing I did before heading upstairs was to get out two birthday cards to send to my friends who would be celebrating in a couple days. I wrote each of their names on the tops of their cards and added a heartfelt birthday greeting before my signature.

What was wrong with my hands? They were shaking. Was I cold? No. These were tremors. It looked like the writing of a 90-year-old woman with Parkinson's disease. I freaked out for a second, then recalled how one of my anti-rejection meds caused tremors. Bummer. Then I smiled and decided to acknowledge it in my card to my friends with some self-deprecating comment. Nothing I could do but laugh about it.

I made my way to the stairs to tackle my climb to the bedroom. It was actually a piece of cake, although a slow walk with two feet on each step, holding tightly to the stair rail. I got into my non-hospital bed just the way the PT had shown me, and Dave took his first stab at propping pillows so I could sleep relatively comfortably. He did a great job.

Before we fell asleep, I grabbed his hand and placed it on my chest. His eyes went wide! He looked at me and said, "I have never felt your heart beating so strongly... and so fast. You feel so alive!" It was the best way to end my first day home and the start of my incredible new chapter! Sleep came easy.

On Saturday morning, a nurse was scheduled to come over to draw blood, walk me through my meds (again) and ensure I knew all the ins and outs of my new daily pill-filled, vitals-monitored, movement-measured lifestyle. I gave myself enough time to make myself presentable.

A shower! My first shower at home in almost two weeks. I did not anticipate how exhausting it would be. I could barely keep my arms elevated long enough create suds in my hair. I had to rest them several times during the time I rinsed out the shampoo and conditioner. As weak as I felt, I could not get out of the shower without shaving.

My one shaky leg was holding me up while I shaved the other. My legs looked so weird. My knees were swollen, I had several bruises, my calves seemed bigger than usual. It was like getting to know a new body. I looked down at my six-inch scar covered in surgical tape; I ran my fingers over the long trails of bruises up and down my arms. My belly was bloated. For the first time, I actually saw the three small horizonal scars where my chest tubes were. Wow! I was a mess. A beautiful, heathy mess. This was my new way of looking at things—reminding myself how lucky I was.

I thought taking a shower was hard? *Oh my God!* Blow drying my hair felt worse than doing a straight hour of lat pull-downs at the gym. My arms were shaking. I kept having to turn the hair dryer off and set it on the counter. At one point, I had to sit down on the toilet to rest.

My next chore was to get dressed. Putting on my panties and joggers was no problem. My bra, on the other hand, was a total failed attempt. As soon as I got it "into position," I winced in pain. What was I thinking? An underwire bra sitting on top of (and slightly digging into) my scar? Seriously? That thing came off after three seconds. I pulled a hoodie over my head and called it good.

I made my way down the stairs—one step at a time. I walked into the kitchen. My mom gave me a look that said, *I'm happy to see you, but I'm still worried, and I will be watching every little thing you do to make sure you don't do too much too soon; I'm your mother and this is my prerogative.* I gave her a good morning kiss on the cheek.

The doorbell rang, and we invited the nurse into the house. We all gathered around the high-top table in our kitchen. We got through the pleasantries, signed a bunch of paperwork, and got down to business. We began by talking through my 16 prescription bottles that equaled 32 pills a day taken at four intervals: 7 a.m., 9 a.m., 9 p.m., and bedtime.

We reviewed what each pill was for, potential side effects, and which ones absolutely HAD to be taken on time, versus the ones that had a little more leeway. She scared me enough that I was totally committed to be on time, every time.

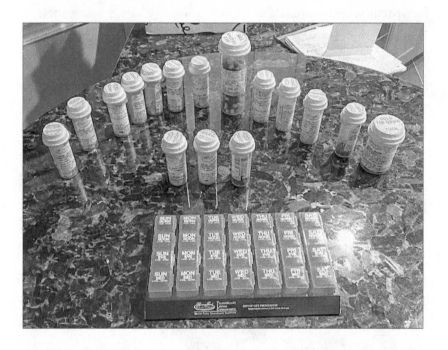

A side effect of one of my meds is diabetes. I was about to learn how to properly prick my finger and monitor my blood glucose three times a day. She told me what glucose number I needed to stay below, what foods to avoid so I could keep my numbers in check, and what would happen if my reading got above 200. What happens above 200? I start giving myself insulin shots, that's what! I thought she scared me with my pill timing. The thought of daily insulin shots truly frightened me, and I had zero interest in going down that path.

I LOVE sugar and sweets and dessert, but not enough to risk daily injections. *I promise I will be a good girl.*

After about 45 minutes of education and veiled threats, we bid the nurse goodbye, and I beelined for the couch to nap. I'm not sure how long I was out, but when I got up, I took my blood pressure and my temperature–things I had to do three times a day. I was getting excited about my first walk. I stood up and did my warm-up exercises. I flipped my left wrist to activate my Apple watch, tapped the exercise icon, selected "indoor walk," and started on my journey.

I walked from the family room through the kitchen, around the dining room table, to the living room, around the chairs, down the hallway, through the kitchen, back into the family room, through the kitchen into the dining room (I walked around the table counter-clockwise this time), made a figure eight around the living room chairs for round two (look at me making it interesting), and back down the hall. I checked my heart rate every couple minutes. It started at 101 and made it up to 120. Seven minutes were up after several laps that resembled my route above.

As I was cooling down, I panicked! I felt a sensation crawling up my insides. *No! Oh shit! I'm going to sneeze. This is going to hurt.* I waved my arms crazily to get my mom's attention. I needed my red heart pillow. They taught me in the hospital that when I was going to cough or sneeze, I needed to squeeze the pillow to my chest to absorb some of the stress. As my mom was scrambling for the pillow, I looked up at the ceiling, quickly sniffed, took in a couple short but deep breaths. I did it! I willed the sneeze away. Disaster averted. Mom was primed and ready to come to the rescue.

I sat on the couch and grabbed my laptop. *Oh boy. Here it comes again.* I looked at Mom and feverishly waved my hand in front of my nose.

She handed me the pillow, and sure enough, "Achoo!" I closed my eyes, regained my composure, and let out an "Owwwwww. That hurt!"

Mom looked at me with great empathy and a bit of parental sympathy pain.

Well...now I know.

I flipped up the screen of my laptop and entered my notes into my newly created 11-tab spreadsheet. Every day, I monitored: my weight, my meds, my exercise, my temperature, my blood pressure, my blood glucose + what I ate, my low and high heart rates, and my stretches. I also had a tab for all my upcoming appointments, I journaled daily, and I kept a list of questions for my doctors. Until this very minute writing this paragraph, I hadn't looked at it since June 30th, 101 days of documentation. Because I'm a dork, I just now added up the total number of entries from each of the 11 tabs — 959 lines of documentation. I guess I needed something that felt like work while I was off for more than three months.

The doorbell rang. It was another delivery. Another box with soup, a ladle, a dishcloth, a bag of cookies, and a bag of dinner rolls. Loving Spoonful was filling up our fridge. It was wonderful! Packages were being delivered multiple times a day. Cards were flooding the mailbox. I made sure to take a picture of each gift and text an immediate "thank you" to each thoughtful person who put a smile on my face and warmth in my soul. At one point, my mantle had seven large bouquets on it, plus other vases full of flowers throughout the house. And as I write this, I'm wearing a pair of fuzzy slippers a dear friend gave me.

The morning of my second day at home, I did something that still to this day stuns me. It stunned me in a scary way back on March 21, but it stuns me in a positive way today. I overcame a fear, a loathing, a deep-seated anxiety to truly see my body for what it is. I asked

Dave if he would take a picture of me in shorts and a sports bra so I could remember where I came from and what I knew I could become.

I posed awkwardly straight-on, turned to the side, then he took a final shot of my backside. It took me hours to actually look at the photos. When I finally got up the nerve, seeing myself was awful and beautiful at the same time. I was horrified but proud. I actually looked the worst, fattest, and most out-of-shape I had ever looked in my life. But on this very day (and the 21st of every month following, when I repeated the photo shoot), I was finally OK with it.

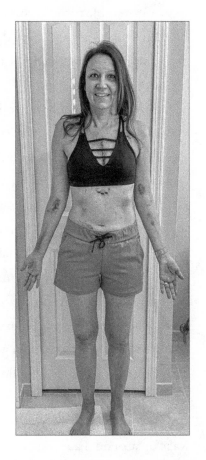

This was the worst of me and the best of me. I made an unconscious decision from that day on to finally relax about how I viewed my body. I realized at that moment how much time, energy, and negative emotions I had wasted worrying about how I looked. And the crazy thing was that at any given time over the last 35 years, I looked a hell of a lot better than I did in this new post-transplant body. But you know what?! I was totally cool with it. I was honestly at peace. I felt liberated. It's like I was able to finally shake the body image demons that had been living inside me for decades.

I was alive! There was way more to me than a flat belly. I was a human vessel that had been given the greatest gift someone could ever receive... and by a total stranger, no less. The scars were worth it. The bruises didn't matter. The bloating meant surviving. This experience was an incredible turning point for me.

I'm guessing that mental exhaustion primed me for another nap–one of the many daily rituals I was becoming very used to, and honestly kind of enjoying.

My first few days home followed a very repeatable routine: wake up, take drugs, go back to sleep, weigh myself, take my blood pressure, check my blood sugar, take more drugs, eat breakfast, document results, rest, take my blood pressure, take my temperature, stretch, do my laps around the house, document results, rest, check my blood sugar, eat lunch, do laps around the house, stretch, snack but not on something sweet (a hard habit to break), document results, rest, check my blood sugar, eat dinner, have something sweet (because I was done checking my blood sugar for the day), do laps around the house, check my blood pressure, take more drugs, journal, document, take more drugs, stretch, then go to bed.

Dave would prop my pillows, I would clumsily crawl under the sheets lying at a 45 degree angle (not on my back, but not on my side, and definitely not on my stomach), fall asleep, and like clockwork wake up around 3 a.m. Ah, the prednisone insomnia.

Chapter 12 – The Revelation

ONE MORNING DURING MY first week home, Mom and I were chit-chatting in the kitchen. My cell phone rang. It was one of my cousins, calling to see how I was doing. I sounded healthier and more energetic than he was expecting.

"How are you feeling?" he asked. "What does it feel like to be home?"

We talked about me being in the hospital, and what that whole experience was like. Out of nowhere, I started talking through an observation I had; it was being shaped as the words left my mouth. This phone conversation truly was the catalyst for me writing this book.

He, like many others, related my exceptional recovery to my state of general good health going into my transplant. As I was hearing this for at least the twentieth time — from nurses, family members, my doctors, friends — I started to formulate a theory around my success. I launched into my diatribe:

"Yes. I was as physically healthy as I could be going into my surgery. I have a strong understanding of nutrition, so I don't have to work at knowing how to eat well. I speak up with my doctors and ask questions about things I don't understand. I am a disciplined person, and I actually want to do everything the doctors are telling me. I have an amazing social network; people are sending so much love and support my way. I am strong emotionally. I have a positive outlook, and

I don't let things get me down. I don't worry unless there is something to worry about. I have inner peace and understand self-care. I've learned not to stress about not working for several months. I've learned to embrace the journey no matter how difficult it will be. I'm made for this kind of challenge."

I wasn't trying to brag. I was just piecing together several key components that I believed made me cut out for this recovery. Then I turned it around to the opposite scenario. This epiphany has since kept me incredibly motivated to help people. And I don't want to just help transplant patients, but it was the transplant patients who were my elusive subjects and my inspiration. I continued:

"It really makes me sad to think about Harold and Frank* (made up names — I never met these guys) who were in the rooms on either side of me in the ICU. *Remember their names; I will bring them up later.* What if they went home to very little support? What if their wives were nags? What if no one called or visited, and they didn't have anyone to lift their spirits? What if all they wanted to do was go back to smoking or eating unhealthy food? What if they didn't feel like taking their drugs some days, or worse yet, weren't focused enough to sort out their 200-plus pills per week? What if they were stressed about money? What if they had no interest in going to cardiac rehab? What if they were ignoring their daily vitals? What if they barely wanted to "be"?

The scenario really bummed me out. On one hand, I felt very validated that I would be OK and would get through my recovery like a champ. But what about others who fell into the less-likely-to-succeed category? If I could take the discipline and education I had, and marry those with other components of my general wellness, could I help them, or more so others like them?

What if I could take my winning combination and get it out into the world to help people make some life adjustments? I don't ever want to be preachy, and I don't want to come across as better than someone else. I don't want to suggest so much change that someone gets turned off and just decides not to do anything. I didn't really know what this looked like at the time, but I didn't want to sit on it without making an attempt to make a difference.

People go through trauma, and it's usually unexpected. Think sudden illness or the death of a loved one. Sometimes a traumatic event is a long time coming, but still a terrible loss. Like a marriage that is falling apart over a long period of time and is doomed to end, maybe when the kids go off to college. We don't live constantly happy lives. We're challenged. We lose jobs, we lose friends, we suffer anxiety and pressure to succeed, we fear COVID, we fear politics, we fear the unknown.

I know a lot of worriers. I know reclusive people. I know people who don't know how to relax. I know people who unhealthily fear failure. I know people in debt. I know people who are struggling with eating disorders. I know parents who live in fear of their kids' poor decision making. The list goes on. You know them, too. Maybe you are one of the people "I know." I have been several of them at different points in my life. I will never be perfect. But I will always try to be better.

By the way, my conversation with my cousin ended a long time before my mind went in the direction of what the latter chapters of this book will include. Please read on through the rest of my physical recovery, and in Chapters 16 and 17, I will take you through my Wellness Widget, which I developed during the months following my surgery.

Sharing my heart health journey has been important to me, and it has been cathartic to relive, but my purpose for putting my words on paper is truly to help others. Just like I had been doing through my work with the American Heart Association, I loved speaking to rooms full of people and was gratified when I knew even just one woman would go see a doctor about something she had been ignoring for months. I thrived knowing that my voice moved people to action. I want to move you to action — if you're ready. We'll pick this back up in Chapter 16.

Chapter 13 – The Recovery

EACH DAY GOT BETTER. In my first two weeks at home, I went from walking slowly around my first-floor furniture for seven minutes, three times a day, to walking outside for 19 minutes, three times a day, at a brisk pace. Well, brisk for someone who had a foreign organ in her chest and was still trying to gain back muscle.

Almost two weeks to the day from when I had my surgery, I was inspired to write to my donor family. My head was all over the place as I tried to come up with the right balance of gratitude and sympathy. I mulled it over, letting phrases and sentiments swirl around in my head. I got off the couch and walked upstairs. I pulled out some card stock from my craft cabinet, grabbed my watercolors, and hand-painted a card using shades of red and hearts. I hand-lettered THANK YOU on the front.

That was a nice distraction, but it was time to put my thoughts to paper. Knowing I was going to struggle, I got out my laptop and typed, edited, omitted, re-wrote, read excerpts to Dave, revised a few sentences, paused, wiped tears from my eyes, went back to my laptop, read the final-final to Dave, and decided I was ready to permanently ink this into the card.

There are guidelines when sending a letter to the donor family. First of all, everything is anonymous. I write the card, I send it to the donor organization in an unsealed envelope, they approve it, they send it to the donor family, and they document if the family accepted or declined it. I would later learn that my family did receive my card.

I am allowed to include my first name, but can't share my age, city where I live, or the name of my surgeon or transplant center. They encourage recipients to include a bit about their hobbies and interests. I could share how long I was on the list or lived with a heart condition. More than anything, the family wants to know what a difference their gift (their loss, really) has made and what future activities the recipient plans to pursue that may not have been possible without my new heart.

I ended my note with this: "Please know that I will never be able to put into words how grateful I am for your gift of life to me — a stranger. I promise you I will wake up every day thankful for what you have given me. And darn it! I am going to finish that triathlon I was training for 20+ years ago."

Other than my wedding vows, and my parents' eulogies that I thankfully have not had to pen yet, this ranks right up there with the most meaningful things I will ever put in writing. This event weighed on me for days. It still does.

I put the card in an envelope, then I put the envelope in a larger envelope and addressed it to the donor organization. What happened after I put it in the mailbox was 100% up to the family. They could send something back to the donor organization, they could ask to learn more about me, they could ask to meet me. They could do nothing.

I had no preconceived notions of how this would play out. My wise dad predicted that it was unlikely that I would hear from them any time soon. They were grieving. Even if my letter made them feel good about the byproduct of their loss, chances of them jumping to celebrate with me were pretty slim. Dad was right.

I also had mixed feelings about wanting to meet them. I didn't have a desire to seek them out. I had a HUGE desire to ensure that they knew how grateful I was. That could be enough for me. If they wanted to meet me someday, I would do anything I could to give them that opportunity. They were in control, and I would be available to them however they did (or didn't) want me to be.

The next day was another emotional one for me. I was sitting on the couch, something I did more often during those few months of recovery than I have probably done in my entire adult life. Dave reminded me that there were dozens, if not hundreds, of text message responses on my phone and Facebook posts that happened while I was in the hospital, particularly the day I was in surgery. It didn't even dawn on me that there would be inbound messages. I was so focused on everything Dave was doing to keep everyone informed.

Oh my gosh! I was a ball of mush when I got done reading from all the different mediums he had used to communicate with people. I was floored to see that my friends were reposting things to their social networks. Literally, people all around the world, including people I didn't know, were praying for me and asking for updates. I found out that within hours of receiving the call that my heart was on the way, my sorority sisters had organized an impromptu Zoom prayer call.

Most common themes in the posts and texts?

Prayers. Warrior. Rockstar. Hugs. Overachiever. Thank you for the updates. You got this! Awesome. Incredible progress. Team Sidlar (I loved this one). Miracle. Inspiring. Incredible.

My friends and family, two weeks after the big event, were melting me all over again. I felt so incredibly lucky! I have THE BEST tribe!

Another thing I discovered while consuming all these amazing well wishes was that some people had asked if they could send flowers. Dave gave a plug to the paper flower company and also suggested people donate to the American Heart Association. One friend decided to up the social media ante and created a pool for what day I would be released from the hospital. If you guessed wrong, you were encouraged to donate. There were also several responses encouraging people to be organ donors. I loved the benevolence and purpose that was being driven by this situation!

I spent at least an hour responding to people individually and through the text groups Dave set up. I felt so loved, and I wanted people to know how much I appreciated every single comment and note of encouragement. I always liked to think I was good about reaching out to people and making them feel supported. This made me feel like such a slacker and truly inspired me to do better for others in the future. Hundreds of people were going out of their way to make me feel special and noticed and cheered up (and cheered on). It was one of my all-time favorite recovery days.

On my tenth day at home, I got some amazing news at my doctor's visit: "You can go out in public, as long as you wear my mask."

I was not vaccinated yet, and I wouldn't be able to get my first COVID shot for three months after surgery. With my severely suppressed immune system, and not many age categories able to be fully vaccinated yet, I had to be extra cautious. Where do you think I wanted to go for my first outing?

"Can Dave and I stop at Costco on the way home?" I asked.

She said yes, "Of course you can go to Costco! Good pick."

I was so excited. I pushed the cart so I had something to hang onto. We went down virtually all the aisles. I managed to stay upright and moving for the full 30 minutes we were there. I will admit, I was absolutely ready to get back in the car so I could sit for a bit. That trip helped me clock 6,383 steps that day. It was my highest number so far! I had my sights set on 10,000!

In two weeks, I went from 32 pills a day to 28. I was able to decrease my three finger pricks a day to two. My lab work was showing that I wasn't flushing my kidneys enough, so I went from my pre-transplant max of 48 ounces of water a day to 64, then 70, then 80. I have constantly struggled with this, and I now drink 100 ounces a day, which still isn't enough some days.

In those first two weeks, I started my weekly ritual of standing lab work — typically five vials of blood each Tuesday immediately before taking my 9 a.m. meds. I also had two more biopsies, which always required a 5:45 a.m. departure from the house and 6:30 check-in. At 7:30, I would get wheeled into the cath lab. As they were pushing me into the room, we would decide collectively which playlist to enjoy. Nine times out of 10 when I'd say, "Anything but country," they would all cheer.

This particular week, as the nurse was prepping me for my biopsy, Dr. Cowger stopped by pre-procedure. I figured since I had a few minutes with her, I would fire off a few questions.

"Can I drive a stick shift when I'm cleared to get back behind the wheel?"

"Absolutely. Sounds awesome."

"What about this weird bump at the top of my scar? Will it ever go away?"

"Most of them do. You should be good."

"Anything you recommend for my insomnia? I'm taking melatonin. What else might work?"

CHANGE OF HEART

"Melatonin is good, and I recommend Benadryl."

"When can I lift over eight pounds?"

"Eight weeks. Your sternum needs to heal. Definitely don't push it. You don't want to be back here getting re-wired."

Then I asked some immunity-related questions about enjoying hot tubs, swimming, being around COVID-vaxxed or unvaxxed people. Then out of the blue she said, "You need to be careful, but as long as you're safe you can even get a tattoo if you want!"

Where did that come from? In my drugged-up state had I told her that Dave and I were planning to get matching tattoos — a triangle of my old heart rhythm, my new heart rhythm, and Dave's heart rhythm? I was so excited to have her endorsement.

Oftentimes asking Dr. Cowger for permission was like going to mom after dad said no. If I were bummed out because one of the other more conservative doctors told me to play it safe, or wait longer for something, I could always play the Cowger card. She was without a doubt always medically sound and never put me at risk, but she also weighed all the factors, including my overall health, and made decisions that were the best for me — medically and as a person who was finally living the life I had dreamed about for decades.

After our brief exchange, she excused herself and said she'd see me in the lab shortly. When they wheeled me in, there was a good 90's mix playing. It was going to be a good procedure. My first observation was of one of the nurse's super colorful tennis shoes. When I complimented him on his cool kicks, we started a conversation about how his last equally awesome pair had recently been stolen.

I gave them a couple friendly jabs about how cold it was in the labs. I asked if they warmed the defibrillator pads up for me (they did that about 50% of the time). Today was one of those days. Dr. Cowger

148

came in, and it was like a celebrity entering the room. The staff just loves her! One of them announced, "And it is my pleasure to present the talented JC!" Her name is Jennifer Cowger. The mood was set. It was going to be an awesome biopsy.

Once they numbed my neck, Dr. Cowger attempted to insert the catheter through my jugular vein. I felt the pressure, then the release. I felt more pressure, then the release.

She said, "Hmmmm... you're pretty dehydrated today."

I responded with a slightly whiny voice, "Seriously? I drank 80 ounces of water yesterday."

And Dr. Cowger's response made my opinion of her jump up at least 10 more points. She said, "Next time before you come, will you please eat a pizza? You need more salt so you can retain that water."

Oh my God! I love her! What cardiologist encourages her patients to eat pizza? She had me perform a couple breathing procedures, and that did the trick. She was in. The pizza suggestion led us to talking about other food and eventually s'mores. We were about to have a warm spring weekend, so we must have all been craving some firepit time. I announced to the half dozen medical professionals standing around me, "If you haven't tried it, you have to promise me you'll put raspberries on your s'mores the next time. You will not regret it!"

Shortly after all the food talk was over, Dr. Cowger announced, "OK. All set. Everything looked good. We'll have your biopsy results in a couple days."

They wheeled me back to the recovery room, the nurse bandaged me up, and I was out the door two-and-a-half hours after we arrived. Time to stop at the bagel shop on the way home for some breakfast. I was starving and needed food to take my drugs!

Later that day, a friend came over — the one who kept Dave company at the hospital when he was agonizingly waiting for my surgery to be over. This friend is also the wife of the genius who came up with the term Kristy 2.0, which we absolutely love and use frequently! The day she came was early April, and the weather was beautiful. We sat outside, mask-free. I wished we could have visited longer, but I still got tired just having to "be on" for longer than about an hour. She was gracious, and before I started fading, she announced that it was time for her to go so I could rest. Bless her!

We took a socially distanced selfie, and although I love that picture, and it is proudly displayed on my refrigerator, it's when I really started noticing, and being self-conscious of, my moon face. Chubby cheeks are a very common side effect of prednisone, a corticosteroid. Inflammation of the face (most noticeable), belly, and knees were most affected. I found this infographic by Prednisone Pharmacist Dr. Megan, when doing some of my Dr. Google research. It was such a perfect encapsulation of all the adverse reactions people can have to this very effective, but often-tough-to-manage drug.

I'm fortunate that most of these side effects either eluded me or were mild, but the fat face made me nuts. I could hide my knees, and no one could see my belly, but it was pretty hard to hide my face. As much as it was deflating to see in the mirror or in pictures, I subscribed to the same philosophy as the rest of my body. It was temporary, and it was out of my control. I actually had several friends tell me it made me look younger because it plumped up wrinkles and smile lines. I started to shift my thinking and felt grateful — it was like receiving free facial fillers!

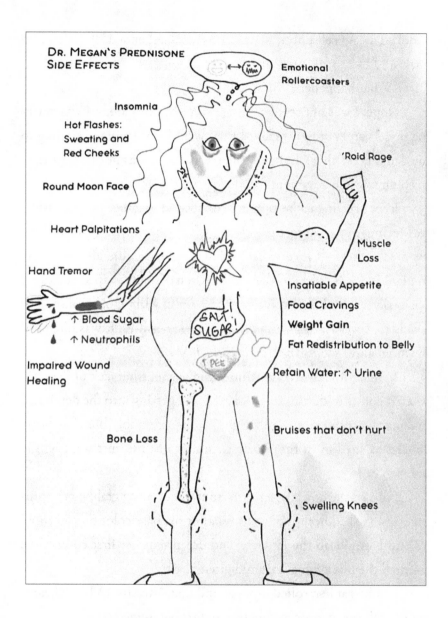

To put an even finer point on how puffed up my cheeks were, I remember being on the phone with my dad one night. He was making me laugh, as he so often does, and the line suddenly went dead.

I looked at my cell phone screen. It said, "Call ended." I dialed him back, and I was still laughing.

"What happened?" he asked.

Nope, I was not still laughing from his funny story. I was cracking myself up because I realized that when I was smiling listening to my dad, my fat cheek hung up the phone. That was not the last time my plump face inadvertently ended phone conversations!

It was getting to be time for my second in-office doctor visit. I was feeling more energetic and wanted to do something special for my medical team. I love to bake. Similar to what I did after my ICD implant in 1999, I decided to make a batch of heart-shaped cookies. I obviously used a different recipe than 20-plus years ago, because all of a sudden, I was staring at five dozen blank canvases. It was fine until my mom and I sat down to embellish them.

Mom and I have a long-running joke about her lack of patience when it comes to decorating cookies. I love getting into the detail and making the cookie look "just right." Mom "assembly lines" as many cookies as she can in the shortest amount of time, just wanting the event to be over.

I placed the bowls of icing in front of her, and I grabbed the piping bags. I asked her if she would slather the base color on the cookies and I would do the lettering and detail. For her first cookie, she smeared the black icing on a mid-sized heart.

I looked at her, rolled my eyes, and said, "Really?" A black heart? I could tell she was processing this and trying to recover.

She covered another cookie of the same size in pink. She held them both up, looked at me and said, "Your old heart and your new heart!" We busted out laughing. I grabbed the piping and wrote "Old Heart" and "New Heart" on the cookies. Look closely!

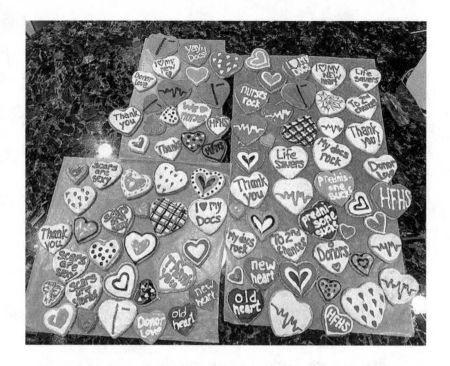

We got a little silly for a while and made cookies that said "prednisone sucks" and "scars are sexy." We graduated to more sincere sentiments such as, "I love my new heart" and "donor love" and "we love nurses" and other expressions of gratitude. Mom hung with me the whole time, even though she asked at least five times if I was really going to decorate ALL the cookies.

A day I had been looking forward to for weeks was my first day at cardiac rehab, April 16, just shy of four weeks after arriving home from the hospital. By this point, I was walking two or three times a day for 30 minutes, and I had hit the 10,000 steps mark multiple times. I checked in for the first of 24 sessions — three days a week for two months.

The rehab specialist showed me how to apply the monitor leads. I was in a small locker room with six other patients all doing the same thing — placing an EKG sticker on their upper chest above their heart and two on their belly. We were all given a little white pouch that tied around our necks and waists to hold the monitor. Two techs sat at the front desk, monitoring everyone's heart rates and exercise intensity.

For the most part, my rehab consisted of the treadmill and a combo recumbent bike/elliptical machine. I wasn't allowed to use the arm bike in the beginning, or anything else that stressed my chest. That had to wait until the tenth week after surgery. Before I got started, they asked me about my goals for rehab. I said, "If there is any way I can run before the end of my 24 weeks, I will be so happy! If it's safe and you think I can, I would love to be able to run again. It's been over 20 years."

I loved rehab. I looked forward to doing something else that was active beside walking the neighborhood or, Lord help me, the first floor of my house. I craved progress and seeing improvements in my physical strength. I paid close attention to my increases in speed, incline, and duration. I planned to be an A patient!

I typically did rehab, plus some other exercise the same day. I was now at the point of mentally "needing" to walk 10,000 steps each day and close all my rings on my Apple watch. Closing my rings meant at least 30 minutes of exercise, standing up 12 times a day and moving for at least one minute each time, and moving for the equivalent of 490 active calories.

I loved feeling so active and alive! Admittedly I was getting a little obsessed. Oh no! Some of the old, workout-crazed Kristy was creeping back in. I look back now and realize how much of my ability to exercise so much each day was way easier when I wasn't working and writing a book.

After three weeks (nine workouts), I was bummed to have to call the rehab clinic and cancel for the day. Looked like I would slip to an

A minus. I was having some gastric issues and couldn't risk being away from a toilet for too long. I texted my nurse to let her know how I was feeling. I was told during my education in the hospital that I had to contact her when anything out of the ordinary happened — fever, cough, headache, diarrhea, shortness of breath, edema, gaining more than two pounds in a day. They told Dave this, and they told my mom this. They were serious!

She said my stomach issues could be any number of things, the most likely of which were a reaction to my drugs or a virus. We made some adjustments to my meds, but for the next couple days, the issues remained, and I was feeling really blah. I spent more time resting on the couch and napping, and my excellent exercise record started waning.

After a couple days, she asked me to go to the lab for some tests. The virus they were worried about could be detected by a blood test, but it took about 48 to get the results. I went in on a Thursday afternoon, but because they needed to monitor the culture for two days, they couldn't send it out until Monday. That would mean I wouldn't have my results for almost a week. That was one long wait!

On Wednesday, I had my regular office check-up with Dr. Cowger. The nurse took my vitals and reviewed my exhaustingly long list of meds to ensure their records matched what I was actually taking. She left, and Mom and I hung out, chipping away at a variety of topics.

Dr. Cowger walked in and said "Hi" to us. She saw me looking at something across the room. She turned to focus on what my mom was holding — a large blue gift bag with tissue and ribbons.

"I brought you something!" Mom extended the bag toward her, and Dr. Cowger rifled through the tissue paper. Mom and I both smiled as she pulled out a box of graham crackers, a bag of marshmallows, a multi-pack of Hershey bars, and... fresh raspberries! She promised me she would make them that weekend.

The appointment was another good one. My recovery was going better than expected. I could never get enough of hearing that! We talked about my recent symptoms, and she suggested a few med changes. At the end of the visit, we got to my list of questions. I always had at least a dozen.

"When can I stop using the red heart pillow when I'm riding in the car?"

She laughed and said, "You're still using that thing? You can definitely ditch the pillow!" Another fabulous milestone.

Later that afternoon, my nurse coordinator called. My CMV (Cytomegalovirus) results were in. I did, in fact, test positive. More than 50% of Americans have been exposed to CMV. Most healthy adults never experience any symptoms. Immunosuppressed people who have it, definitely know they have it. I was now one of the unlucky ones. An adult with a healthy immune system who has CMV, will test with a cell count of 137 or less. My cell count was 26,000! No wonder I felt like shit (pun intended).

When heart transplant patients are diagnosed with CMV (about 30% of us are), we need to be admitted into the hospital for IV treatment. They wanted to get me in right away, but the cardiac unit of the hospital had no beds. I waited two days and finally got a room on Friday evening. Due to heightened COVID cases, I was not allowed any visitors. They started my IV immediately.

I actually felt pretty well. The biggest bummer about being in the hospital that particular weekend meant that I was going to miss the American Heart Association HeartWalk. I had been raising money for weeks. A family-and-friends team of 11 people were meeting on

Saturday morning at 8 a.m. Everyone else showed up and walked in my honor. They sent pictures and words of encouragement. I still felt really good, so I made it my goal to walk 3.1 miles through the halls of the hospital. I did it in three segments, but my Apple watch houses proof that I, too, did a virtual HeartWalk that day.

Shortly after clocking my final mile, one of the nurses came in to tell me that they were ordering a colonoscopy for Monday.

"You'll need to prep tomorrow," the nurse said.

I had had a colonoscopy before, and the prep honesty wasn't that bad. I was up for the task. Most of Sunday, I wasn't feeling great, so I wasn't very hungry anyway. I think I had a Styrofoam cupful of beef broth, a lemon ice, and a cup of Jell-O, not the gross protein stuff. At 6 p.m., they brought in my colonoscopy prep. It was not what I was expecting. What I had used before, a Dulcalax/Miralax combo, had been very tolerable.

But the nurse did not walk in with my preferred cocktail. She brought in something called GoLytely.

"You'll drink it with water," she said.

"Can I drink it with Gatorade?"

"Sure, but we don't have any."

Dave to the rescue! Because I had heard from a friend how awful GoLytely is, I needed something to mask the flavor. Dave went to the store, bought me four, 32-ounce bottles of Gatorade, drove 20 miles to the hospital, and met my nurse in the lobby.

I mixed my cocktail and started drinking around 6 p.m. I was supposed to consume half by midnight and the rest by 3 a.m. I was able to stomach the first quart, no problem. I started slowing down around midnight, but hadn't quite consumed my 64 ounces yet. It was so awful! A few swallows, and I would gag. I slept on and off and tried to drink little bits at a time. A nurse came in around 3 a.m. and said:

"You're way behind on your consumption. You HAVE to finish it by 6 a.m."

I thought that would be doable. But at 5:30 a.m., I still had at least a quart to go. I was texting Dave, telling him — actually complaining — about how I just couldn't finish it. He switched from texting and called me, attempting to convince me to "suck it up, Buttercup" and finish it. He threw out the cruelest comment during that call, and I will never forget it.

"Kristy, you're not being an A patient. You're being a D patient!"

It about killed me to hear that, but you know what? I didn't care. It didn't motivate me this time. Certainly not enough to want to finish it. At that moment, I was OK with a "D." He sweet-talked me into drinking more. I told him I would, but it really was meant to be more of a platitude.

We hung up, and the nurse entered my room. She picked up the container, and held it up to eye level to see how much I had left. She looked at me and very sternly said, "If you don't finish this in the next ten minutes, we will reschedule you for tomorrow, and you have to do this all over again today."

That did it. A-patient Kristy was back. (Even if I were just bullied into it.) I swallowed four more back-to-back servings. I proudly slammed the gallon container down on my bedside table. I pulled the covers up to my neck, gagged, then threw up all over myself. *Lovely!*

The nurse cleaned me up, checked that I had indeed finished my neon yellow drink, and confirmed that I was cleared to have my procedure at 11 a.m. Everything went off without a hitch. I was officially diagnosed with CMV colitis, as they had suspected. I would now be taking pills five times a day — adding my CMV meds to dinnertime. I was allowed to leave the hospital the next day, just in time for my brother to arrive from San Francisco! *Hooray!*

It was wonderful seeing Marty. Due to COVID, it had been almost a year to the day since I had been with him last — the day we left California to move back to Michigan the previous May. We hung out around the firepit, we had the entire Michigan family over, we ate great food, and we spent time with an old friend whom neither of us had seen in more than 30 years. I was self-conscious meeting her again. I was sure all she was going to notice was my fat face. I took a picture of her with Marty, and she took one of Marty and me.

I sent the sibling picture to Mom. True story: she thought the woman standing next to Marty was his friend. She didn't even recognize her own daughter! *Damn moon face!* I did allow myself to laugh about it — eventually.

The next day, Mom and Marty left. This was a bit short of the required 90 days of having two caregivers, but I was doing so well. Docs cleared me to have only one caregiver. I was driving on my own (no red heart pillow under the seatbelt strap), I was running my own errands, I was seeing more people, and I was going out to dinner (outdoors).

Much like thanking my medical team and my donor family, I was in another predicament of having to find the right way to thank someone when there really was no proper way. I did the best I could expressing my gratitude to my mom. I wrote a heartfelt card, verbalized my appreciation to her every way I could, gave lots of hugs, and bought her and her significant other a dinner certificate at a lovely restaurant in Florida.

Not only had she been with me for more than two months, but she had also been away from Richard for that same amount of time. I was forever grateful to him for letting me steal her away for so long.

Chapter 14 - The Normalization

AND NOW THERE WERE two. Dave and I were back to being a normal couple in our own house. I missed my mom, of course, and we began talking multiple times a week by phone. But life was beginning to get back to normal.

Things were looking up! I was now down to monthly biopsies. I had had seven up to that point, all with great results and no signs of rejection. I was down to 21 pills a day. I no longer had to check my blood sugar. I was averaging about 11,500 steps per day. I was drinking 90 ounces of water daily. My weight was steady. My CMV numbers were coming way down. I never expected to feel this great, this quickly.

The following weekend we received much-needed massages. I was finally able to lie on my stomach and enjoy the full experience. Our massage therapist came to the house, and Dave let me go first. As she kneaded my back, she commented how my right side, which was usually very stiff and tense, was much more relaxed; it was my left side that seemed more stressed.

"No surprise," she said, "considering all that part of your body has just been through."

When the magnificent massage experience was drawing to an end, I asked her, "Did you detect anything else unusual about my body this time? Was there anything noticeably different?"

I was so awed by her answer.

"Your left side just seemed lighter. I don't know how to describe it. It was like it was... less full."

Of course! My massive, oversized, diseased heart was no longer taking up all that space in my chest cavity. Feelings of gratitude filled my now smaller heart.

I was back at rehab after an almost three-week break. It felt good to be on the treadmill again, but I did have to back down on my speed and intensity at first. After a few sessions following my CMV break, I was checking in and one of the specialists said, "I heard you wanted to run! I think today is your day!"

I get chills thinking about it, even now. I was excited. I was nervous. I was scared.

Then I remembered there was nothing to be scared about. That habit will need to be broken. For 20 years, running equaled v-tach, which equaled passing out, which equaled getting shocked, which led to progression of my disease. *That disease is gone!* Nothing to fear. Easier said than done, but *LET'S DO THIS!*

I did my normal, 10-minute warm-up. Remember, my new heart has to increase slowly to allow the adrenaline to speak to my brain to tell my heart to speed up. After 10 minutes, the specialist came by and asked if I was ready. I smiled nervously (although she couldn't see it under the mask I was required to wear). She bumped the speed up to 4.8 and away I went. She gave me the thumbs up and yelled over to the desk to tell them to record my numbers.

As soon as she turned away from me, my eyes welled up with tears. I was so incredibly happy. I willed myself to not let those tears spill over onto my cheeks. I tried to think of something other than what this really meant. This was validation that Kristy 2.0 was everything I hoped she would be.

I was able to suppress the tears. The specialist looked back at me. I gave her a wave and a thumbs up. I ran for a minute and walked for four, and repeated that sequence several times. It was hardly anything a real runner would get excited about, but it was such a great start for me. I finished my treadmill session after 40 minutes, did my elliptical thingy, turned in my monitor, and started heading for the door. One of the other specialists caught my attention and said, "Way to go, Kristy! You ran today!"

It was all I could do to get out beyond the threshold of the door so no one could see the real tears. As soon as I got to the hallway, they came in a sudden wave, rolling right down my face while I sniffled and wiped my eyes. I was smiling, but couldn't stop crying. I got into my car and pulled myself together so I could drive home.

During my six-mile drive home, all I could think about was running. *I just ran!* My body liked it. It didn't revolt. My heart rate didn't elevate to 250 bpm. I didn't pass out. I felt great.

As I was turning onto our street, a half mile from home, I was suddenly ugly crying. I was laughing and crying at the same time. I pulled into the garage, walked into the house, and started blubbering and blabbing like an incoherent child. Dave saw me and panicked. I now know he thought someone had died. Hardly... I was so alive! What came out of my mouth next was something like,

Sniffle, sniffle, "Running..." inhale, "20 years..." exhale, "Rehab..." sniffle, snort, "So happy..." inhale, "Oh my God..." exhale, "I'm sorry, I'm fine..." more ugly crying.

Dave pulled me into his chest and just let me get it all out for a good five minutes. The left sleeve of his t-shirt was soaked. He understood. He knew how badly I had wanted this back in my life. When I was done, he looked me in the eyes, smiled, kissed me, and said, "Oh God. You're not going to make me run with you, are you?" We laughed. He pulled me close again, reassured me, and reinforced that he was truly happy for me. If you didn't catch it, Dave hates running.

Knowing that rehab was close to the end, I was feeling a bit anxious about increasing my strength, flexibility, and cardio on my own. I asked around at the rehab facility if they knew any local rehab therapist who also did personal training. They didn't, but said they would check around.

Not one minute after the question came out of my mouth, I remembered that one of my sorority sisters is a personal trainer AND used to be a cardiac rehab specialist. I mean, c'mon. How did I not think of this before now? She lives in Illinois, but who can't do just about anything over Zoom these days?

I contacted her, and after a couple catch-up conversations and consultations, the contract was signed and we were off! Not only were her workouts perfectly structured for me, but she gave me my confidence back. When she told me to do chest flies, I would hesitate and say, "I don't know if this is good for my chest."

She would very kindly and confidently fire back, "You're chest is healed. It's been almost four months. It may feel tight because you haven't used it this way, but you are good."

And yes, indeed, I was.

When it came time for squats, still my least favorite exercise, I hesitated. When I had ARVC, I was not allowed to do squats or lunges. Much like running, they engaged my large muscles in a way that would cause my heart rate to elevate and potentially throw me into v-tach — that super-fast, super uncomfortable and potentially deadly — rhythm. I did squats, and guess what? I was fine. She was one of the absolute highlights of my physical recovery.

I finished rehab after my 24 sessions. It was June 30. I was returning to work the following Tuesday, right after the Fourth of July weekend. I spent the last few days wrapping up some personal projects. I had been doing some watercolor painting and making greeting cards. I decided to do a little hand lettering to put the final touches on some of my cards.

My tremors were unpredictable. Some days I was totally fine; others I would have the dropsies all day, continually missing the correct letters when typing on my phone, and writing could be really embarrassing.

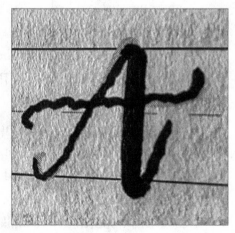

Unfortunately, this was one of those days. Darn drugs. I picked up a notebook to give a few letters a shot, just to see if I could control my pen. After producing this, I quickly set my watercolors back into the drawer and called it quits.

That night, we went out to dinner with friends. It was a gorgeous summer night, and we ate outside. As I was scanning the crowd, Dave gave me the sign to look behind me. There was Dr. Lanfear, having dinner with his family. I hadn't seen him since right after my surgery. I felt like a star-struck fan wanting to tell Bono (my all-time-favorite artist) how much his music meant to me over the last 35 years. But this wasn't music; this was my life! I wanted him to know what he meant to me. And equally as important, I wanted his family to understand how meaningful, and impactful, and life-changing his work is.

I tried to make myself small and quiet as I sheepishly approached his table. "Dr. Lanfear? I'm sorry to interrupt."

He turned and looked at me. Not the kind of "looked at me" I was expecting. I think I was hoping for him to jump out of his seat with a big smile and give me a huge hug. Obviously, I was out of context. He didn't expect to see me at a restaurant. That's why he didn't recognize me.

"It's Kristy, I mean Kristen, Sidlar." My eyes were welling up with (happy) tears.

He immediately stood.

"Can I hug you?" I asked.

"Yes."

As his family was looking at us, he introduced me and explained that I was one of his recent patients. Then he said to me,

"I hardly recognized you. You look great. So healthy. Wow!"

In my head, I immediately went to: *Right...my moon face. My cheeks are so fat, he couldn't make out my features.* In reality, he was sincerely telling me how healthy and vibrant I looked. I know this because he mentioned it to Dave later. *Whew!*

I took this opportunity to walk closer to the table. I looked directly at his wife and said, "Your husband saved my life. I am so grateful. I honestly don't know how to thank him. Knowing how hard he works, I'm sure it's not easy for you, but please know that what your husband does really matters."

I made eye contact with each of his kids and smiled, willing them to honor what their dad does for a living.

Dr. Lanfear and I caught up for a few minutes one-on-one so I could tell him how I was feeling, how my work-outs were going, and that I was training to run a 5K, and how great Dave had been. I could have gone on and on, but I wanted to be respectful of his time with his family. Dave entered the scene for a couple minutes, then we all said our goodbyes. I told him I'd see him at the hospital one of these days. Lord knows I was there enough!

Dave and I enjoyed my last few days off, celebrated the Fourth of July, and I readied myself to return to work. I was so excited to go back — back being defined by working from my home office like most of the rest of the world was doing in July of 2021. I started a new role, still at The Mom Project. I felt a bit like a celebrity; everyone was so kind and welcoming and politely curious and supportive. Truly they had been all along.

My first day back featured a virtual happy hour (I drank sparkling water) with my old team and my new team. It was such a great reconnection. One of my colleagues asked if, after a full workday, I was exhausted. The question was lost on me. I felt fine. Then I remembered how I felt 20 years ago after my ICD procedure. A few hours at the office left me exhausted. Now that I had had almost four months off, was working out religiously, sleeping like a champ, and really feeling like life was pretty back to normal, I had no reason to be exhausted.

In the evenings and on the weekends, I was running more. Shortly after I returned to work, I joined a Facebook group called Heart Transplant Survivors. It was a fantastic resource as I was still navigating recovery. I was also able to offer some of my own experiences and perspectives to other members.

One of the group posts announced that a running race was coming to Detroit. I loved the name of it: Women Run The "D." It was an all-female event with a 5K, 10K, and half marathon. I decided I needed a goal. I signed up and told a friend who is a long-time runner. She said she'd run it with me. I was really excited at the idea. Then I thought: *No way I will be able to run the full 5K, let alone run at her pace. I'll need to walk/run. I don't want to hold her back.*

Before I could say anything, she said, "I'll run it WITH you. I'll go at your pace. I'll run alongside you the whole way. This is for you!"

If I could have hugged her through the phone, I would have. I continued training with my sights set on September 12 — six months after my transplant. Dave even ran with me a few times while I was training. Again... Husband of the Year. Once I started doing longer running intervals, he politely bowed out.

About a month after signing up for the race, I saw a post on the Heart Transplant Survivor site that led to one of the most emotional events of my entire heart journey. Someone posted about meeting their donor family. I chimed into the thread, congratulating her, and expressed a few details about my own transplant. I stated that I didn't have any details due to the laws in Michigan.

Years ago, someone in the Ann Arbor area received a heart. The recipient's family was told the age and the sex of the donor immediately after the transplant. That same week, the recipient's family read in the newspaper about a prominent figure in the local community who died — same age, same sex. They put two and two together. This scenario bred a very uncomfortable community situation and created a policy change. Doctors in Michigan hospitals are no longer allowed to share donor information with their patients. All information needs to go through the donor organization, and as far as I understood, that information couldn't be released to me for one year.

Someone in the Facebook group encouraged me to call the donor organization and ask. She lived in Michigan and was able to get some information about her donor. I picked up my phone, Googled the organization, dialed the number, and made my request to the friendly voice on the other end of the line. She transferred me to a coordinator who asked me a series of questions.

I was fully expecting for her to hear my transplant date and tell me I needed to call back at the one-year mark. I was absolutely stunned when she said, "OK. Here. I see it. Yes. Your donor was a 37-year-old female."

I couldn't believe what I was hearing. She just told me that I am living with a heart given to me by a woman who was likely in the prime of her life. I was suddenly so sad. I held myself together while I asked a few more questions: "Can you tell me anything else? Where she's from? Am I allowed to know the cause of death?"

She responded sympathetically with, "All we are allowed to tell you is the age and the sex. The only other thing I can tell you is whether or not they received the letter you wrote. We keep track of whether the family accepts or rejects correspondence from the recipient. Let me see. Yes. They did receive your letter. That's great!"

We talked for a few more minutes. I thanked her profusely, and as soon as we said our goodbyes, the tears began rolling down my cheeks. I got up from my desk, searched the house for Dave, and tearfully recounted my conversation. It was a profound moment. Later that night, I shared the experience on my Transplant Tribune Facebook page:

> I am a ball of emotions right now. I just found
> out the age and sex of my donor! It was a 37YO

female. I know nothing else — no location, cause of death, or family situation.

On a whim, I called the Michigan Gift of Life office. I thought I wasn't able to know for a year from my transplant date, but she was able to tell me on the phone. She recommended that I write another letter to the family to let them know how I'm doing now.

"Heart donor families tend to LOVE knowing about heart recipients more than any other organ," she said.

I feel really strange, but very happy, finally knowing. I'm sad again for the family; this definitely re-opened that reality. Above all, I am so thankful!

That conversation took several days to sink in. Emotions were swirling every which way. It's still very vivid in my mind, and it continues to fuel me to live the best life I can with this precious gift. I continue to place my hand over my heart every day and give thanks. I am now able to be a little more focused on whom I'm giving thanks to.

The weekend of September 12 was finally upon us. Race day. My mom and Richard were in town, sadly for my uncle's celebration of life. My Uncle Chip was yet one more member of my mom's side of the family affected by heart disease. He was a super healthy, at-the-gym-six-days-a-week, incredibly young-looking, 77-year-old when a massive heart attack took him from us.

At 6:30 a.m. on Sunday, the four of us and my friend drove down to Detroit for the big event. It was a cool, cloudy morning. I was wearing my Donate Life hoodie, and donning Donate Life (green) and Heart Association (red) shoe charms on my laces. Every time I looked down, they reminded me what I was running for.

We met up with my friend, checked out the booths, soaked in the energy from the other runners, and killed time before lining up for our 5K. The half marathon and 10K runners would take off before us.

For about eight minutes before our event was about to start, I broke off on my own to start walking at a brisk pace to get my heart rate up. I perform best when my rate gets up to about 120 bpm before running. I got to where I wanted to be and made my way back to all the runners who were lined up. We ended up having to wait a good 10 minutes during announcements over the loud speaker, and I jumped in place trying to keep my heart rate elevated. Finally, the gun went off, and we were running! It was exhilarating!

My girlfriend was the perfect running partner. She kept with my pace. She walked when I needed to walk. She empathized when I said, "OK no more talking for me. Gotta breathe."

I had a little friendly competition with a couple other walk/runners who were doing intervals like me. I had my sights on a couple whom I wanted to be sure crossed the finish line after me. Sorry, my competitive spirit was getting the best of me again.

I could see the finish line. We were less than a minute away. My friend faded back and pulled out her phone. She snapped a couple of pictures of me, then switched over to video. She caught me running all the way to the finish line.

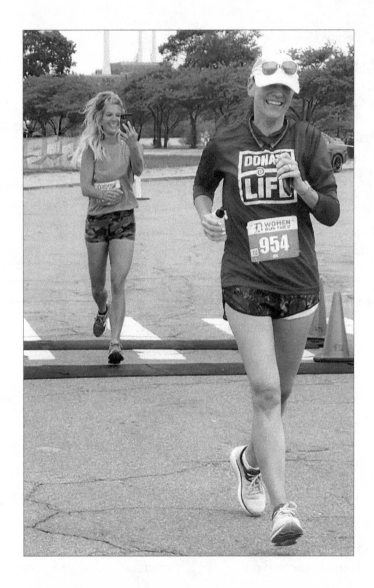

When I was about 100 yards out, the announcer said:

"All right, guys. Next... eyes on the finish line. We've got my friend Kristy Sidlar here."

I instinctively raised my hands over my head and pumped my fists.

"Six months ago she had a heart transplant!" she said. "Her first 5K in 20 years, and she chose to do it here." Her voice was quivering. Even she was moved by the magnitude of that moment.

I crossed the finish line all smiles, arms still over my head.

The first face I saw was Richard, then my mom, then Dave. My mom and I embraced, both in tears. I grabbed Dave and hugged him, then pulled away. I was having a bit of a hard time catching my breath. I composed myself, then walked to Richard for a hug. Finally, I saw my friend, still with her phone in her hand, gave her a huge embrace, and whispered, "Thank you."

What a day! I will never forget it. And I don't think I will ever feel those same feelings again. There truly was nothing like it. We were home by 10 a.m. I took a nap and got ready to honor my uncle's beautiful, meaningful life. Talk about a day with an enormous swing of emotions.

My second 5K came a few weeks later. Then I shifted my focus to diversifying my training; my decision was made to complete a triathlon. That elusive event that slipped through my fingers in 1999. Right around the time this book will hit the shelves, Spring of 2022, my mom and I will be crossing the finish line together in a sprint triathlon... hand-in-hand.

Chapter 15 - The Release

ALL THROUGHOUT MY RECOVERY, I had my eyes set on the prize of finally being able to get back on a plane and travel "home" to California. We missed our house, we missed our friends, and I absolutely missed my NorCal family. We couldn't wait to get back on the trails and attempt some elevation this time, as I had been relegated to the flats pre-transplant.

Getting the all-clear from my docs was music to my ears. I was triple vaxxed, and as long as I masked up on the plane, washed my hands, and didn't touch my face, they felt totally comfortable with me heading west. Because my biopsy results had been so solid over the last six-and-a-half months, they even told me I could skip November and do my next biopsy when I went back to Michigan for Christmas.

A couple weeks after 5K number two, Dave and I packed up and headed back to California. The last time we were in our house had been May 8, 2020 — 17 months prior.

We were beyond eager. We loaded up the cats, filled more suitcases than we needed to, got a ride to the airport from our nephew and his fiancée, and headed back to my happy place — the San Francisco Bay Area.

The most exciting thing happened the morning after we arrived. We started our day with one of our local favorite Sunday rituals:

going to the farmers market in our little downtown. We got dressed, walked out the front door, and for the first time since living in that house, I looked at our 47 steps and smiled ear to ear! I knew I could tackle them this time without having to stop two thirds of the way up.

I glanced at Dave, looked at the stairs, and headed straight up. Not only did I feel great, I was bounding up each step faster than ever, even outpacing Dave. I'm competitive, after all, so I made a point to stay ahead of him. And, of course, I was pumping my arms in the air when I got to the top! I was hardly even out of breath.

Getting my lab work done, which was still a weekly affair, became one frustration after another. One lab lost one of my critical vials. It's probably still floating around the mail system. One lab forgot to draw another key sample, even though I had asked the phlebotomist four times, "Can you please read to me everything you're drawing today? Can you please walk me through the stickers on each of the vials? Can you please confirm everything you just drew? Did you get my CMV and Tacrolimus levels?"

Sure enough — they screwed it up.

We finally got everything squared away when there was a bit of a panic about a month after I had been back in California. It was a Friday morning, and I was on a work call. My mobile phone rang. "Nancy A" was displaying on my screen. Nancy is my nurse coordinator. I texted back:

Sorry. On a work call.

It's important. Did you take your meds yet?

Not yet. Call you in 2 minuntes.

I ended my Zoom call and hit redial on my phone. I was feeling anxious while waiting for Nancy to answer. One ring was all it took before I heard,

"Kristen?" It was NOT Nancy. It was Dr. Lanfear.

Now I was definitely feeling concerned. I tried to sound cool: "Hi! What's up?"

He shared that the local lab lost my Tacrolimus results again. My Tacrolimus is the drug I take to stave off rejection. During year one, it was important that my level stayed around 10. Two weeks before this, it had been 7.9, and last week it had dropped to 4.7.

The 4.7 had freaked me out a bit, but my nurses said the drop was likely a combination of moving my med times from the Eastern Time Zone to Pacific, even though I did it very gradually. Another possible cause was that if I weren't getting my blood drawn exactly 12 hours from my last dose, my numbers could be affected.

I did admit on the call when a nurse told me about my 4.7 reading that I had been drinking some wine since I had moved back to California. Her reaction was quite severe.

"What? You're drinking wine?"

"Yes. I was told as long as I didn't drink within two hours of taking my Tacrolimus at night, I was OK to have a glass or two."

Her tone became very stern, and she asked, "Who told you that?"

My answer in my head was *Dr. Mom, of course.* Yes. Dr. Cowger had given me those instructions during one of my latter visits.

"You should not be drinking in your first year." This nurse scared me enough to stop that! (Mostly.) We ended the call with her making another adjustment to my meds to get my "tacro" level back up.

Anyway, back to my conversation with Dr. Lanfear. Because we were approaching the weekend and because my last two readings were going in the wrong direction, he needed to get results today. As much as I wanted to counter him with how many work meetings I had that afternoon, I stopped myself and said, "Sure I can go to the lab right now."

Nancy arranged for me to go to the pre-eminent medical center in the Bay Area. I got a call from the local coordinator and was sitting in the lobby of the hospital lab within 40 minutes of that first call from Dr. Lanfear. It was a little past 12 hours since taking my meds the night before, but we would at least have an answer with relatively accurate readings that afternoon.

Finally, at 10 p.m., the results were in. I picked up my phone, opened the My Chart App, pulled up the portal, and typed in my password. Of course, my fingers missed the right keys (darn tremors). I tried again. Success! Tacrolimus was in bold at the top of the list. I tapped it. 9.7. All good. *Whew!* I was back on track.

As relieved as I was to read this beautiful number, I was a little bummed to think that maybe there was something to this not drinking thing. Mind you, I am not much of a drinker. I never have been, and I always had to play it safe with my ARVC. But here I was, living in northern California, knocking on Wine Country's door, and I had a cellar full of wine that was calling my name. It was hard to resist.

A few days later, I was in for a HUGE treat. I was finally going to see my Dad and Linda for the first time in 550 days! I had last been with them shortly after COVID started, and right before we were to fly back to Michigan in April of 2020. We had all sat in my dad and Linda's living room wearing masks, six feet apart and trying to feel remotely normal as we caught up for a few hours.

This time was going to be a whole different experience on so many levels. I wanted to speed the whole way. My parents live up the Sonoma Coast and the last hour of the trip is one hairpin turn after another. Most of that part of the trip is up on the cliffs of Highway 1, and much of it without guardrails. Speeding was not in the cards that day.

Pulling into their driveway after the two-and-a-half-hour drive gave me serious butterflies. I was beyond excited to hug them both. Like all good parents, as soon as they saw my headlights coming toward the house, they were on the porch willing me to get out of the car. It was the sweetest feeling — the best hugs I had gotten in way too long.

Being with them for a couple days, and knowing I would be back the next weekend with Dave and my brother Marty, made the energy in the house like nothing we had experienced... maybe ever. Us being together eradicated so much of the isolation and anxiety and uncertainty of the last 18 months of COVID and not being able to see each other during my recovery. It was a heavenly few days for all of us.

I returned home and back to my new routine. The fabulous lab facilities were my new go-to and everything remained under control. My labs were coming back on target, and I continued to remain steady, even with the occasional two ounces of wine once or twice a week.

It was approaching Thanksgiving and I finally felt the urge to write that second letter to my donor family. I started with:

> To my precious donor family,
> First of all, I think about you and your daughter/sister/wife/mom (?) daily. I literally put both my hands over my heart and give thanks to her and all of you each morning (and usually several other times during the day). I celebrated my 53rd birthday a couple weeks ago and often wish I knew what

her birthday was so I can celebrate her on her special day too.

When I first wrote to you, we were all in a state of huge change — yours much more emotionally painful than mine. Mine filled with gratitude, but so sad for your family. Amongst your grief, I want you to know how much your gift of life has meant to me.

I continued sharing with them how well I had been doing and how much "my" new heart has allowed me to accomplish things I had only dreamed about for the last 20 years. I again expressed how inadequate I felt trying to thank them for their gift. I signed off, inserted a photo of me crossing the finish line from my first 5K, put the card into an envelope (unsealed) and addressed the larger envelope to the donor organization. As of this writing, which is 50 days after sending that card, I have not heard back.

That same night, I went for my first proper swim since training for the triathlon in 1999. My gym offers adult novice swim classes. It was the perfect fit for what I wanted to accomplish. I knew how to swim, but I needed some expert tips on how to be the most efficient. I absolutely loved the class. You could not have wiped that smile off my face that night if you tried.

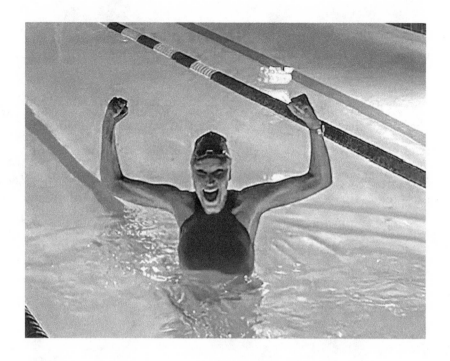

Thanksgiving and Christmas came with some very special opportunities for me to reflect on what an incredible, full, miraculous, challenging, and rewarding year I had experienced. Although I just spent almost 50,000 words putting my feelings and experiences into this memoir, I really can never fully express how 2021 has changed the trajectory of my life. I want nothing more than for this book to inspire and impact and affect change in others' lives, too.

I spontaneously coined a phrase when I was a guest on my first podcast. The host had brought me on to talk about my transplant experience. Her last question was an invitation to share any final thoughts I wanted to impart on her listeners. I thought my response would be a fitting way to close these chapters before shifting gears to my wellness segment:

"To me, SCARS ARE STORIES. That took me a while to understand... that a scar is not a bad thing. It's a reminder of, for me in my case, a second chance at life."

You may not ever go through an organ transplant (I'd say your chances of that are probably really slim), but you will be challenged. And whether your scars are physical or emotional or financial, or a result of any other kind of adversity, those scars, if recognized and accepted in the right way, can propel you to tell your own 2.0 story.

Please join me in these final two chapters as I share tips and advice on how to invite change into your life through practical tools so you can become your best self.

Chapter 16 – My Wellness Widget

IF YOU RECALL FROM Chapter 12, "The Revelation," I described the contrast between: 1) the way I have approached total wellness; and 2) the life choices of my fictitious ICU brethren Harold and Frank. There is not a week that goes by (really almost daily), that I don't think about that scenario when I make choices. I evaluate if they are the best choices for me and compare them to poor choices. Believe me when I say they aren't always the easiest choices, and many times aren't even close to perfect choices. I envision the upside, and I weigh that against the downside.

We all make thousands of choices a day, so I'm not talking about whether I do or don't pick up my cat at a certain moment or grab the red grocery bag versus the one with the pelican on it. I'm talking about health choices, life choices, and what-matters choices.

During the course of my recovery, I gave wellness choices a lot of thought. Not only do I think about Harold and Frank, but I think about other people in my life who want to "do better." This drives me to live as an example to help others make smart, long-lasting decisions, discover new approaches to living more healthfully, and to take action to create real change, not just a temporary, feel-good fix.

Throughout most of my career, both as an employee and as a manager, I have always been acutely aware of how best to develop people. I have also observed the wrong way to do it. It has always made me nuts when leaders or general company policies have expected more out of their workers without giving them the tools to be successful.

As an early-career salesperson, I would be told to be more strategic. I was expected to be better without any guidance that would elevate my skills and get me to the best result. I have heard employees across various companies being told that they need to be more efficient. No tools or automation were provided to improve output. I have seen recruiters who were given new stretch goals for an increased volume of candidate contact. No training was provided to further develop their skills and refine their approach to make their calls more effective.

In all of these scenarios, there was little to no improvement. The company failed the employees, and in turn, the employees failed the company. I have made it my mission as a manager and now as an author to provide tools and ensure no one is left to figure it out for themselves. I can't guarantee 100% success, but I will do everything in my power to give you the equipment and ideas. Success requires discipline, and it requires identifying and understanding what may be undermining your success.

In these last two chapters, I ask for you to be open to adopting some practices that can contribute to living a more fulfilling life. They may seem hard. Stick with me. They may seem easy. I ask that you stick with me through these areas as well. Sometimes ease can be deceiving. A change can be easy to adopt, but harder to sustain.

Megan Call of University of Utah Health states in a 2020 blog, "Behavior change is complicated and complex because it requires a person to disrupt a current habit while simultaneously fostering a new, possibly unfamiliar, set of actions."[1]

I believe that the greater your desire to change, and perhaps the intensity of the negative impact if you don't, drives a lot of our motivation. Motivation breeds discipline. Discipline breeds success.

The last few months have allowed me to reflect on several dimensions of wellness that I truly believe have contributed to my successful, speedy, and sustainable recovery. I'd like to take you on a journey through my Wellness Widget.

This chapter includes the general concept and definitions. I will exemplify positive and negative scenarios of each of the wellness dimensions, and we will work through some self-reflection. This may even lead to journaling if you're into that kind of thing.

I'd love for you to close this book, holding onto some practical ideas that you can immediately start infusing into your daily living. Maybe some of you will have a life-changing challenge in the near future, and you want to get ahead of it for your own healing. Maybe you know you have an Achilles heel in reaction to certain things life throws your way. Maybe you have always struggled with a dimension of your wellbeing that you just haven't been able overcome. Or maybe someone in your life is struggling and you want to be the best supporter possible. Maybe my Wellness Widget approach will bring some things to light for you!

The Wellness Widget

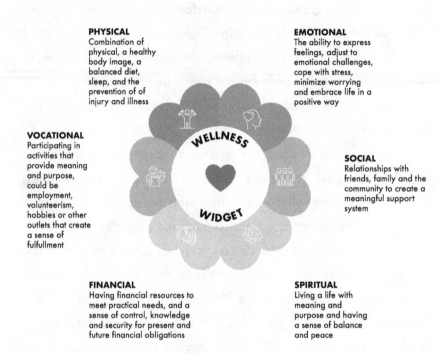

PHYSICAL
Combination of physical, a healthy body image, a balanced diet, sleep, and the prevention of of injury and illness

EMOTIONAL
The ability to express feelings, adjust to emotional challenges, cope with stress, minimize worrying and embrace life in a positive way

VOCATIONAL
Participating in activities that provide meaning and purpose, could be employment, volunteerism, hobbies or other outlets that create a sense of fulfillment

SOCIAL
Relationships with friends, family and the community to create a meaningful support system

FINANCIAL
Having financial resources to meet practical needs, and a sense of control, knowledge and security for present and future financial obligations

SPIRITUAL
Living a life with meaning and purpose and having a sense of balance and peace

I have seen many versions of "your best approach to wellness" since self-care and holistic health have been in vogue. In my quest to keep things simple, I have taken the areas that have been most meaningful to me and boiled them down to six.

I spoke with Kristi Piehl, an Emmy-award winning reporter and host of the *Flip Your Script* podcast, a few months after my transplant. Her response to my explanation of the Wellness Widget was such a great summary of how we can take these six dimensions of wellness and use them as a guide to comprehensively improve our health.

"You're never 'good,'" she said. "You can always get better. You can always get a little more healthy. You can always have a little bit more financial stability. So, it's this ongoing, lifelong evolution that continues, and as we go into different seasons of our life and relationships, they look different. But I think there's this mindset of 'Check. Done.' No! Because each of those areas can always be moving — forward or backward — and because, like so many things in life, standing still means backwards."

She continued: "...With so much of wellness, people go to health or they go to weight or they go to clothes size. I love that you're talking about these six things that are connected, but maybe not always in the same conversation."

Spot on, Kristi Piehl!

Before we get started, I have to admit (or disclaim) that I am not a psychologist or a spiritual leader or a financial advisor. What I share with you is experiential. My approach to life has created the joy, satisfaction, fulfillment, and ability to pay it forward that I can only hope impacts you and those around you in some way.

Physical Wellness

This seems to be a pretty obvious wellness dimension. Physical health is such a critical foundation to all the other aspects of our wellness. The National Institutes of Health describe physical wellness this way: "Positive physical health habits can help decrease your stress, lower your risk of disease and increase your energy."[2]

Here's my definition: the combination of physical activity, a healthy body image, a balanced diet, sleep, and the prevention of illness and injury.

I believe physical wellness starts with having a strong foundation for exercise, movement, and ways to maintain our physical vessel. Diet is another key component. Of course, diet is different than diets.

I do not believe success comes from diets. It comes from a heathy, sustainable, lifestyle diet. I do believe very strongly in the motto: all things in moderation.

Most people would consider me a very healthy eater, but I am by no means a perfect eater. I will, more often than not, reach for a salad or a healthy snack option. But I will rarely pass up the opportunity for a (small) bowl of ice cream, a (little) cookie or *one* piece of candy.

Could I be a more perfect specimen of the chemical components of a healthy person? Yes, probably. I do, however, feel confident through my weekly bloodwork that my chemistry is fine. I am able to live with a good balance of satisfying my cravings, which keep me from feeling deprived, and with choosing healthy options, which makes me feel physically and mentally satisfied.

In researching other wellness models, one thing I found missing from the physical definitions was having a healthy body image. As you know by now, this was a very big struggle for me throughout my life. We can be physically fit, which is a good thing. We can have discipline around our exercise and our eating habits, which is a good thing. In my case, however, those were not managed to healthy proportions. It was important to me to elevate this component when encouraging people to look at the full wellness picture.

In my case, eating well and exercising was not always done in a healthful way or for the right reasons. I think that's why calling out a healthy body image is so important for me. I want to shine a light on this for the world. Women, in particular, tend to have, or have thrust upon them, unrealistic standards. I have found that being hyper-focused on what society or other women deem as the definition of health and beauty, can have a negative, harmful effect.

I could probably write a whole book on body image, but I won't hijack this chapter with this single topic. I will say that I learned over the course of way too many years that I wasted an incredible amount of energy worrying about how I looked, what others might think about how I looked, and whether or not somebody was looking at a particular part of my body. As I reflect on my fruitless fretting over multiple decades, and particularly when I look back at pictures, I actually looked pretty darn good. God! All that fuss for nothing! I'm relieved to be (mostly) rid of all the negative self-talk and unproductive worrying.

Shifting back to overall physical wellness, my biggest lesson has been the realization that your physical health can be taken away at any time. In my case, it was taken away slowly over a period of time and revitalized based on a major life event. Other people can have their physical wellness depleted in an instant and have a slow, painful fight back. But as people told me over and over and over during my recovery, the reason I bounced back so well was because I had taken care of myself over the long haul and across all areas of wellness.

I mentioned earlier that my husband Dave is a pretty terrible sleeper. He has taken proactive efforts to get to the bottom of why that is and what he can do about it. He has endured sleep studies, he has read books, and has listened to expert podcasts. He has researched supplements that he is now taking. He has purchased an Oura ring that has helped him understand the triggers for restful and restless sleep. He is now very conscious of how to be a better sleeper. He made a commitment to learn and to make improvements.

Lastly, it is important for us to focus on prevention of illness and injury. As an inherently impatient person, I am prone to skipping warm-ups, stretches and cool-downs. When I started running after my 20 years off, I overlooked preparing my body. I did experience sore knees and some other early onset injuries. As much as I wanted to push through because I was so excited to get back to running, it was important to stop, evaluate, research, and act on other professionals' advice. Stepping back so I could leap forward was the best thing I could have done.

Let's walk through a couple of scenarios to get you thinking about where you are in your physical health journey and what potential actions you can take to make improvements that work specifically for you.

For Your Reflection

I strongly encourage you to take time with the reflection sections of this chapter. Consider starting a journal and focusing on the areas where you wish to improve. Recording your thoughts and desires is a great way to stay focused, track your progress, acknowledge setbacks, and commit to adjustments.

Another thing to consider with each of these six dimensions of wellness, is that you may choose to focus on only one element or each of the subcategories. For example, with physical wellness, you might pull out the balanced diet component and focus solely on that. Or you could take the time to reflect on multiple areas such as physical activity, body image, and prevention of illness. These could each become part of your journey to better overall physical health. Let's give it a try!

1. Think of a time when you wanted to challenge yourself, but didn't take the initiative. What got in your way? How did that make you feel? Could you use this experience to fuel better results in the future?

2.   Think of a time when you accomplished something you set your mind to with respect to your physical health. What contributed to your success? How did that make you feel? Can you devise a plan that will allow for replication of this success?

The goal with all of these exercises is to be honest with yourself. Dig into the why. Understand the pull either away from or toward something negative or positive. What drove you to make the choice you made? How can you replicate the great choices, and how can you alter your approach when you didn't get the result you wanted?

I encourage you to expand on these exercises. You can likely create some of your own reflection questions and translate them to other areas for improvement.

Emotional Wellness

My definition: the ability to express feelings, adjust to emotional challenges, cope with stress, minimize worrying, and embrace life in a positive way.

Much like body image was an area I uniquely added to my physical wellness definition, I found a void in many of the definitions I read for emotional wellness. I didn't see an emphasis on minimizing worrying. I have very strong opinions about worrying. Frankly, I think worrying is a huge waste of time and energy. Let me put a finer point on that. I mean needless worrying, which I define as having anxiety about something that is out of our control. I can feel concern, and I can wish that a situation doesn't result in a negative outcome, but I believe pure worrying when it can't change anything, is useless. I'm not sure who or what I get to credit for this realization early in my life, but I am so grateful for the ability to bypass this negative emotion.

As I mentioned in my prologue, I am an optimist. I know many people who are realists, and I know many people who are pessimists. I choose optimism, not to put my head in the sand or to overlook reality. But a positive mental attitude and outlook can be prophetic. Going through life feeling positive impacts so many things beyond one's mental state.

Worrying is only one of the many emotional elements I reference. Other areas, like being able to adjust to challenges, cope with stress, and express feelings are all part of a healthy mental state. If I reflect on much of my adult life, although you wouldn't know it by how many times I referenced crying throughout my book, I have often had challenges expressing my feelings, particularly when, in my view, they portrayed me in a negative light or showed me lacking toughness. I was a very infrequent crier because in my mind, crying was a key indicator of weakness. I still don't love doing it, but I have moved well past my inaccurate, lifelong judgement of tears.

I distinctly remember a conversation with my stepmom when I was in my early thirties. I have exceptionally close relationships with all of my parents and always saw myself as a very open, communicative member of the family. She pointed out a personal characteristic that has stuck with me ever since.

She said, in a loving, want-to-be-helpful way, "It feels like we get the same Kristy everyone else gets. We're your family, and we love you, and it seems as though you are guarded around us."

What she meant was that I had a block to truly opening up to the people closest to me. She didn't see me getting vulnerable or sharing what may really be going on in my life. She was right. If there were ever something happening that could be perceived as negative, I feared judgement. I felt a need to be portrayed as perfect. Well, of course not perfect, so let's say positive. I feared that if I spoke of something challenging or if I talked about a negative scenario and was able to turn it around without anyone knowing, I could save being perceived as tarnished. As I write this, I'm probably a therapist's easiest target. I have had my share of therapy, and I do really value it!

These revelations are the direct result of someone guiding me to be better. We all have opportunities to grow, and if someone or something doesn't force you to see it, you're in charge to change it yourself. Here are a few exercises to prompt emotional growth.

For Your Reflection

1. Think back on a time when you held back on expressing your feelings. Did you regret it? Maybe you would have had the opportunity to make someone's day who really needed it. Or did it have a positive outcome? Maybe holding your tongue when you wanted to tell someone how you really felt, was absolutely the right decision. How can you adjust or recreate your reactions to situations to uplift yourself or others in the future?

2. Think about a time when you worried about something out of your control. How did it affect you? Looking back, would you change how you dealt with the situation? Looking forward, how can you plant a trigger to divert worrying in the future?

Social Wellness

Definition: Relationships with friends, family, and the community to create a meaningful support system.

I have always considered myself to be a social creature. My first grade report card stated, "Kristy is an excellent student, but she is a bit too social." I love interacting with people, I crave learning from them, I seek out interesting exchanges, and I like to think I give back to people through my outreach and engagement with them. I never want to be stagnant, and what I gain from and give to other people through social interactions is very important.

For many people, reading that previous paragraph is paralyzing and painful and absolutely off-putting. Introverts take a very different approach to social engagement. Extroverts gain energy through outward stimulation and social interactions. Introverts focus inwardly and recharge by spending time alone. In our very social society, introversion can have a negative connotation, but it is a perfectly healthy personality trait. In fact, it can be a very efficient way of navigating the world. They often have a low threshold for small talk, so cut through "the bull" and find ways to enjoy more deep and meaningful conversations.

Approach aside, it is very important for our overall wellbeing that we are connected to friends, family, and community to truly live a fulfilling life.

As a social creature, it has always been easy for me to make connections and find ways to bring people into my life, both for my benefit and for theirs. I have, however, during many phases in my lifetime, involuntarily retreated from social interactions by overemphasizing other areas of my life.

This tends to happen when I put too much energy into work and volunteerism. This has created a negative imbalance and left people close to me feeling ignored. Of course, working and volunteering included elements of social behavior that satisfy *my* need for social stimulus, but pouring so much energy into these areas of my life has hindered positive interactions with the intimate social circle of my family and friends.

This was amplified when Dave and I lived in Singapore. The 12-hour time difference made interpersonal interactions difficult. I also worked too much when we were in Asia and was too reliant on technology when I did actually make time for human connections.

After three years of mostly text messages and emails, I had all but abandoned my ability to be physically present and available to my family and friends when we moved back to the U.S. We had been warned before leaving Singapore that repatriation is harder than expatriation. I thought that was a ridiculous statement until the reality of re-entering life with people I hadn't spent physical time with for almost three years truly was an effort. I wrote down goals for my re-entry. Focusing on being more present with friends and family was my number one priority.

Volunteerism, when done in moderation, has been a very positive example of my social wellness. It checks the community box, and it also gives me great joy to give back and impact others' lives. It provides me with a meaningful support system while I simultaneously become part of a support system that is bigger than me and provides for others. Through volunteerism, I have met some of my closest friends and have been one small but significant part of impacting change. Some of the ways I can feel good about volunteering include:

creating awareness, raising money, increasing women's confidence, and giving children shining moments in an often-underwhelming life.

For Your Reflection

1. Are you an introvert or an extrovert? How do you think that impacts your social wellness? Would pushing yourself more in one area or another create a different experience for you? Maybe think of a variety of scenarios where being more introverted or extroverted would make you feel more satisfied or allow you to positively impact others in your life.

2. Think of a time when you pushed yourself out of your comfort zone with respect to your social engagement or inward focus. Did you get the result you were expecting? Was it positive or negative? Would pushing yourself in that direction again be worth the effort to get another positive result?

Spiritual Wellness

Spiritual wellness is the newcomer in my life, at least the way in which it has manifested within me today.

My definition: living a life with meaning and purpose and having a sense of balance and peace.

I am definitely in a constant state of development, and spiritual wellness is probably the area where I still have the most work to do. I struggle with organized religion, but I've learned to distinguish spirituality and faith from church and the biblical God. Through a

spiritual lens, I found a lightness and peace that I continue to culti-
vate throughout my life.

My spiritual journey has been a labyrinth. I credit my impression-
able personality for the path I've taken. It took me a long time to figure
out who I am spiritually, and because I have been all over the map, I
feel very confident that I've landed in a place that is best for me.

I've flexed from being an atheist, to being a born-again Christian,
to realizing that faith and peace and spirituality are very unique to
each person. In my view, my right answer is likely not someone else's
right answer. What gives me the most joy about my spiritual journey
is that I have grown to be very accepting of others' beliefs, and that
has given me a real sense of peace. I strongly encourage you to open
your minds, minimize judgement, and see spirituality in others as
something to respect.

There was a time when my beliefs were very polarizing to others
in my life, particularly in my family. I was stubborn, others didn't see
things my way, and that frustrated them... and me. I pushed, because
I believed I was right. As my beliefs have shifted, I have learned to live
by the motto: if what you believe makes you feel fulfilled and happy
and safe, and those beliefs are not hurting you or others, I am 100%
supportive.

This realization was not only liberating, but it has given me so
much joy to appreciate, support, and engage in conversation that
makes everyone feel heard and encouraged. The opposite scenario,
when not seeing eye-to-eye with someone else's beliefs and practices,
can be extremely and unnecessarily detrimental. I can finally say I
truly feel happiness for everyone whose religious or spiritual practices
make them feel happy. This realization is exhibited in many parts of
my life. Empathy is such a powerful tool.

When looking internally at how I can improve my spiritual wellness, I have turned to meditation, yoga, and quiet introspection. When I first started practicing each of these, particularly meditation, I was pretty awful. I did not try all three of these at the same time, thankfully; that would have been a recipe for a triple failure.

Yoga came first. I fought meditation way longer than I wish I had. And quiet introspection has come to me since my transplant. I have a very active mind and always thought I couldn't shut down, so why try? And when I did finally make the commitment, I had tremendous difficulty focusing. But like many things, it took practice and discipline, and through this I have found that these practices have created an abundance of peace, quiet energy, and focus that I never would have thought could be so instrumental in my overall wellness.

For Your Reflection

1. Think back to a time when you felt you had a strong sense of purpose. How did you channel it? Have you been able to maintain it? How can you infuse a sense of purpose into your life daily? How could you replicate this sense of purpose to help yourself and others more regularly?

2. Think of a time when you were feeling a sense of turmoil or experienced trauma. What did you do to bring yourself peace? Is this a practice that is easy or hard for you? Can you reproduce the steps you took and make it a habit?

Financial Wellness

My definition: having financial resources to meet practical needs, and a sense of control, knowledge, and security for present and future obligations.

Wow! The hardest part of this definition for me, and I think most other people, is control. That's a big ask, especially in a world where so many of us love and crave instant gratification!

What has financial wellness meant to me? I have learned so many valuable and often painful financial lessons throughout my life. I grew up in a single parent household. Granted, my dad was very present and financially supportive; my mom was very frugal and taught us the value of saving. I will admit she was much better at teaching than I was at practicing.

Like many 20-somethings, I lived paycheck to paycheck and saved little. Thank goodness for some good advice and the ability to save some money through 401k's and IRA's. Like my mom, I was divorced in my late twenties. I was single and living in San Francisco, one of the most expensive cities in the U.S. I wasn't quite living paycheck to paycheck, but I was also very prone to feeling the need to buy what I wanted when I wanted it and put myself into a bit of debt. I was saving more because I was making more, but I still lived beyond my means.

To a person who loves buying based on instant gratification, getting out of debt is one of the hardest and least gratifying efforts. This was the point in my life when I finally heeded my mom's advice. I wish it wouldn't have taken me so long, but I did finally get there. It was a turning point that made me realize the value of a little sacrifice now for some great rewards later.

A piece of advice I would like to give from personal experience is the value of engaging a professional to manage your finances. I have had a few financial planners during my adult life, and I have seen multiple methods of money management. The absolute best thing that Dave and I did for our financial stability was to engage one single financial planner who looked at all our finances holistically.

Instead of managing our 401k's ourselves, plus having short-term savings through banking institutions, plus investing in mutual funds for retirement, plus buying stocks for short- and long-term gain, we hired someone to manage our entire portfolio. He reviews our goals on a regular basis, he understands and documents our retirement interests, he takes into account our long-term healthcare needs, he asks questions about our lifestyle, he assesses our comfort with or aversion to risk. He has 100% visibility to all our dollars. Because of this, we have never been in a better position or had a better handle on how our money is working for us.

When flipping financial comfort to financial struggle, I think we'd all be hard-pressed to come up with a more stressful scenario than being in a negative financial situation. I remember the early days of my parents owning their own business. They were struggling to make payroll, which would mean letting down their employees. The service they were providing occasionally and unexpectedly had intermittent breaks in delivery, and that negatively impacted their customers. I learned through those struggles that there is really not much worse stress in the world than financial stress.

If we work hard enough at it, if we make sacrifices, and if we can get ourselves in a position to survive the unexpected, our stress levels will go down and our financial wellness will improve. This, however, is much easier said than done. Life can turn on a dime, and the less stressful way to deal with that is to have prepared. How does it feel when you absolutely need money, and then look back on a time when you "needed" instant gratification? What if you had made a more future-looking decision?

Another aspect of financial wellness that has come more easily later in life, but has always been important for my financial wellbeing, is giving back. Even when I was younger, I knew the importance and satisfaction of being able to give when others need it more than I do. In most cases, this was exemplified by giving to charities and organizations that needed funding. Even small contributions when I didn't have a lot to spare meant a lot to me.

Another way I have more recently looked at giving back, comes from a quote my friend shared with Dave and me more than 10 years ago. It has stuck with me ever since. When tipping a worker or giving money to someone in a situation where there is an evident need, oftentimes we will debate in our own minds what amount to give. It's easy to default to the lower end.

I don't know this person. They won't know that I was debating between $5 and $10. I'm still probably giving more than they might get from others.

What our friend imparted on us was, "C'mon! That extra few bucks is not going to make a dent in your wallet. Don't you think they need it more than you do?"

That quote always rings in my head when I even remotely think about holding back on a tip or a donation. And it always makes me smile when I reach a little deeper.

For Your Reflection

1. Reflect on how you feel when you are in a financially stable situation versus when you are financially stressed. What are some things you've learned about yourself? What changes, big or small, can you make to reduce the number of financially stressful situations in your life?

2. Have you been in a situation where you or a loved one has needed to make financial sacrifices? Can you describe the sense of accomplishment when the situation was resolved? What choices or changes can you make in your own life that would minimize the sacrifice or stress?

Vocational Wellness

I have to admit, I struggled a bit with what to call this wellness dimension. I considered occupational, I considered pastime, I considered livelihood. None of them perfectly fit. And I'll be honest, I'm not sure vocation completely hits the nail on the head, but this is the umbrella I am using for this wellness dimension definition: participating in activities that provide meaning and purpose, which could be employment, volunteerism, hobbies, or other outlets that create a sense of fulfillment.

Vocational wellness has been a mainstay throughout my life. I don't do well with idle time. Finding ways to occupy myself translates to social experiences, educational improvements, intellectual stimulation, getting my creative juices flowing, and of course, a paycheck. I have often suffered from an overabundance of vocation and have at times lost my sense of a healthy balance. I love filling my life by doing things I enjoy. I am often over-stimulated, and this can cause my other dimensions to get out of whack.

I knew prior to my surgery that this would be the first time in my entire life that I would have a four-month break. The amount of downtime I was about to experience actually scared me. I was being presented with the opportunity to not work and be allowed to do nothing but focus on myself. Obviously, the majority of that four months was spent on physical improvements, but I knew I would have free time and got ahead of it by figuring out ways that I could fill up my months off. I took up watercolor art and designing greeting cards. It was very fulfilling. This vocation falls into the hobby category, and I do believe everyone needs one or multiple hobbies.

For many people, the key vocational category that occupies the majority of their time is paid work. Most of us need a job for the majority of our lives to meet our basic needs. I'm sure you know the quote from Confucius: "Choose a job you love, and you'll never have to work a day in your life."

Many of us are not as fortunate to love our jobs to the point where it doesn't feel like work. However, if you can find something you truly enjoy most of the time, it will be as close to vocational wellness as you will likely ever experience.

The biggest factor I see in vocational wellness is using your time wisely and creating a purposeful, fulfilling life. When someone retires, that means the paid work stops. That can be devastating for many. Just because someone retires, doesn't mean they stop being fulfilled. Some people do struggle with retirement and suffer from lack of usefulness once they stop working. Until the day we die, we need to find ways to fill our time and create that sense of purpose and fulfillment.

For Your Reflection

1. Do you have a job, hobby, or community outlet that makes you feel especially fulfilled? How would you feel if you had more time to pursue it? Can you create a plan for your life that will allow you to pursue more of what you love?

2. Do you have a pursuit you share with someone else? If so, how does that play into your social wellness? If not, how do you feel about pursuing your vocation independently? What rhythm can you get into that allows for you to get the most out of your vocation, profession, hobby, or livelihood?

Chapter 17 - Your Transformation

MY GOAL IN FOCUSING on these six dimensions, my purpose in writing this book, and my long-term vision for my readers is that I can positively impact others. I want to inspire people to think differently, focus on health and wellness, and to not settle for the things that are hindering them, holding them back, or blocking their ability to be fulfilled.

A secondary goal for me when inspiring people to take action and make even slight tweaks to how they live their lives is to have their actions impact others. I am a big believer in the "pay it forward" concept. I want you to make improvements because you read this book, and I want those improvements to allow you to positively influence the people around you.

As much as I try to surround myself with positive people, I have lived my life hearing from, being around, or experiencing negative people with detrimental attitudes and cranky dispositions. I think it's safe to assume that when these people are in a negative state, not only do they feel miserable, they're usually making the people around them miserable, too.

You may recall, I referenced in my prologue that I can sometimes appear a bit Pollyanna. Bear with me as I express an attitude that might fall into that category. I often envision a scenario that may seem far-fetched. That scenario is simple, it's hopeful, and it's something I wish for constantly. I want a domino effect of positivity. I want one person's positive energy to infect another person with positive energy.

Here's my ideal scenario. Nothing would make me happier than to think "Cranky Carl" makes a positive change that makes him feel better. And by Carl feeling better, the people around him feel more positive about Carl. Carl has made a few small changes in his life that have made him more interesting, desirable, and easy to be around. His positivity inspires the people in Carl's life to not only want to be with him more, but to make small changes themselves. Those changes are noticed by their friends and family and the inspiration chain continues.

Wouldn't the world be a better place with more positivity and less conflict? I love being an optimist, and I love having a positive outlook. I've strived to live my life with the glass half full because it makes me feel good, but truth be told, there is an external joy to my optimism. When I know I can make someone else feel good, or I can inspire someone to be better, or I can use an experience that should have dragged me down, but actually lifted me up, I focus on channeling those experiences into others.

I have a strong desire to entice someone to change their mindset and flip their way of thinking. Maybe that flip is for a few moments, maybe it's hours, days, or a lifetime. If I can be the catalyst for someone becoming a better person for themselves and ultimately for those around them, I have accomplished what I was put on this earth to do.

Whether you find **one thing** from my Wellness Widget to hone in on and elevate to something you are committed to working on for the long-term, or if you saw **a little something in each** of the dimensions, I challenge you to keep working at what you want to improve.

Much like the employee training example I gave at the beginning of Chapter 16, when people aren't given tools or they are given a directive that is too broad to actually act on, the chance of success is low. Pick one thing! And then pick another. And then pick another.

To come at this final chapter with a sense of solidarity, let me tell you what my one thing is for each of the six dimensions. I am publicly committing to making different choices when it comes to each of these areas. I choose to do this for me, and I choose to do this to pay it forward to others. I have printed out my Wellness Widget graphic and hung it on my wall in my office. I have added to it each of the commitments below.

Physical — Move more. I work out regularly and I do enjoy a multitude of activities that keep things interesting. However, as I look at my sphere of physical wellness, especially since I sit at a desk most days, I want to find ways to get more movement into my life. My new balance board and stand-up desk will play a part in this.

Emotional — Say, send, or write something that makes someone feel good. I love to share with others something positive about how they look, how they performed, and what they accomplished, but I can always do more. I will work to write and send at least one more note of encouragement daily.

Social — Pick up the phone. We live in such an electronic world. I spend the majority of my work week on video and phone calls. It can be exhausting to make one more call at the end of the day or on the weekend. I promise to progressively increase my volume of voice-to-voice interactions.

Spiritual — Meditation. I love it, but have gotten away from it since going back to work, writing my book, and training for athletic events. This practice is coming back into my life! Tip: two apps I love are Insight Timer (free) and Inscape (paid subscription).

Financial — Be more involved in our financial plan. This one makes me cringe to commit to in writing. I have never enjoyed looking at the details, and it takes a lot to get me to contribute to decisions about how we save for the future. I usually default to whatever Dave suggests. I know it frustrates him that I take a backseat. I will be a better partner in this area.

Vocational — Choose work, hobbies, and interests that fuel my other dimensions. It's one thing to enjoy what I put my energy into, but I have decided I want to channel that joy into improving my other wellness dimensions. For example, I love to make greeting cards. Can I tie that into my emotional wellness goal of sending a word of encouragement to people? In my workday, can I move more during or between meetings and calls? Absolutely, and I just set up my TRX bands in my office so I can do a few exercises when I need a break.

Richard O'Connor, psychotherapist and author, wrote in his 2015 book, *Rewire,*

> The bottom line is that there are powerful forces within us that resist change, even when we clearly see what would be good for us. Bad habits die hard. It seems as if we have two brains, one wanting the best for us and the other digging in its heels in a desperate, often unconscious, effort to hold on to the status quo.[3]

As true as this statement is, it is never too late to try to be on the winning side of the battle of the brains. Change is hard, but the reward can be great. I opened this book with my desire to be on the side of winning. Yes, I am a competitive person, so winning has always been in my sights. Winning, however, does not have to be associated with competition.

Win at wellness! Win at being the best version of yourself. Win at making others around you have a better experience because of their interactions with you. Your winning can impact their winning, and so on, and so on. In my wildest dreams, I could only hope that my advice to you and my approach to overall wellness could make even a small change the world. But what if it could? What if YOU could?

The challenge is on, and my money is on YOU!

Chapter 18 – Ask Me Anything

GETTING A HEART TRANSPLANT is not a run-of-the-mill procedure you hear about every day.

Approximately 3,000 people in the U.S, or .001% of the U.S. population, receive a donated heart each year. That's the equivalent of seven people in the entire state of Alaska annually. And even in a heavily populated state like California, .001% is equal to fewer than 400 heart transplant recipients annually out of a population of 40 million people. These statistics fuel my sense of gratitude, especially considering that more than 100,000 people are on the heart transplant list in the U.S. each year.

Because heart transplantation is so uncommon and because I have been asked dozens of questions from friends, family, colleagues, and curiosity seekers, I decided to wrap up this book with an FAQ to give you a deeper view into the transplant experience.

By far, the most common question I have gotten is:

"Do you know who the donor is?"

As of this writing, I still do not know who my donor is. I have contacted the family twice through the donor organization. It is up to the donor family to reach out to me if and when they are ready.

"Do you know the age and sex of your new heart?"
Yes. My donor was a 37-year-old female. I do not know her exact birth-day, although I would very much like to. I will not know that unless the donor family contacts me.

"How do they match a heart?
Does it have to be from another female?"
The two main criteria for making a donor heart match are blood type and body size. I am a small-framed female and best matched with other people my size whether they are male or female. A large man's heart would not have been a great match. Although with how enormous my heart had gotten, I clearly had enough room in my chest!

"Do you feel different?"
Heck yes, I feel different! It's like night and day! I think oftentimes when I'm asked that question, people want to know if my heart feels different or if I "feel things" from the donor.

"Have you picked up any personality traits or characteristics
from your donor, or do you recall any memories from her?"
Memories, no. Personality traits, I don't think so, but I suppose that is up for debate. I have developed a few new behavioral characteristics. I am more emotional, but I tend to attribute that to the magnitude of what I've been through and my openness to feeling the often-over-whelming gratitude of my gift. I am also a bit more direct and unwill-ing to put up with pettiness. Again, I think my life perspective has changed a bit and I want to spend my energy on what matters most.

"Why so many drugs? What do they do?
Do you have to be on them your whole life?"

I take drugs for so many reasons. The biggest is for immune suppression. My natural immune system wants to fight off my new organ. If it did, that would cause rejection of the heart. I was taking anti-virals, anti-bacterials, and anti-fungals, but reduction of my steroid has allowed me to stop taking those. My steroids and immunosuppressants create other issues, so I have taken blood pressure medicine and cholesterol medicine. I also take several vitamins and supplements, because my drugs weaken my bones, lower my magnesium and potassium, damage my kidneys, and myriad other side effects. After year one, assuming I am stable, I will take about 15 pills a day for life (and only twice a day). I'm done with the five-times-a-day routine.

"What have been the worst side effects?

There have been two. The tremors and hair loss are both side effects from my anti-rejection drug, Tacrolimus. The tremors come and go. Most of the time they are just annoying, but the worst time is when I'm cold. I can go from feeling slightly chilled to shivering uncontrollably. The hair loss was a tough one because I have thin hair to begin with. I think I dealt with it pretty well. Much like my swollen belly and fat face, I knew it was temporary and I couldn't control it, so I just dealt with it the best I could. It wasn't worth stressing over, since it was out of my control.

"Any beneficial side effects?

This is really weird, but as a result of one of my anti-rejection drugs, I no longer have underarm hair, and I barely ever have to shave my legs. It's awesome!

213

"When will your immune system go back to normal?"
I will take immunosuppressive drugs for life. At the two-year mark I should be back to having a relatively normal immune response. That said, we will always have to strike a balance of warding off infection and preventing rejection.

"What's a heart biopsy like?"
A heart biopsy is performed to monitor rejection. The experience of getting a biopsy is different for different people. They don't bother me. I don't even take sedation anymore; it never did anything for me anyway. Some people get extremely anxious and require max sedation. I don't like to look at the monitor when the catheter is doing its thing in my chest cavity. Some people really like to see what's going on as it's happening. I have asked the team to show me the tools they use, and I even got to see the teeny-tiny tissue samples they took from the wall of my heart.

"What does it mean if you show rejection?
You don't need another new heart, do you?"
My immune system detects my new heart as a foreign object, just like it would a virus, and can start to attack it. Many patients experience some level of rejection in the first year. I have not so far. Rejection is always a risk, which is why it is so critically important that transplant patients do everything possible to stay virus- and bacteria-free, and maintain a high level of overall health. Unfortunately for me, female recipients, particularly with female donated hearts, are at the highest risk.

Rejection rarely means the recipient needs to get another new heart. I am constantly monitored through bloodwork and biopsies. I also need to be concerned if I ever start experiencing the symptoms

I had when I was in heart failure: shortness of breath, swelling of my feet and ankles, sudden weight gain, feeling weak and tired, and a few other new symptoms like fever and a drop in blood pressure.

"What is your life expectancy?"
Wouldn't it be awesome if we all could know that? Research, and conservative estimates say a heart can last on average 12 to 15 years. I have done a lot of research on this subject, and as you can imagine, that data is based on history from the 50-plus years of heart transplants. The 12- to 15-year statistic includes mortality rates of the first hearts in the 60's and 70's. I have talked to many people who are 20, 25, and even 30-plus years out from their transplants and still doing amazingly well. I plan to be around for a very long time with this new ticker of mine!

"What was the first thing you remember during your initial recovery?"
My first memory was within hours of being moved from the OR to the ICU. I was hot and I was trying to "communicate" that to Dave and the nurse.

"What did they do with your old heart?"
The team performed some pathology on the diseased heart and disposed of it. Sorry I can't give you a more sensational answer! It didn't end up in the Heart Hall of Fame or anything.

"What is the physical/medical state of the donor?"
A donor heart comes from someone who has been declared brain dead but is still alive. The donor family must consent to donating the organs.

"For how long can a heart remain viable prior to transplant?"
Four to six hours. The heart has the shortest window of all organ transplants. Because of this, the location of the donor heart plays almost as much of a part in matching as do the blood type and body size.

"Were you ever considered 'dead' during your surgery?"
No. Machines kept me alive during the time when there was no heart in my body.

"How did they keep you alive with no heart in your chest?"
Tubes were inserted into my chest so the blood could be pumped through my body with a heart-lung (cardio-pulmonary bypass) machine. Once my blood was completely diverted to and pumped by the machine, they removed my diseased heart.

"How much pain were you in after surgery?"
You may find this hard to believe, but I was in very little pain. They gave me morphine for several tube and IV removals, but I never did request any pain medication during the general course of my recovery. I expected a lot of pain going into the procedure, but fortunately, I was disappointed! I have had bruised ribs before, and I was fully anticipating that unbearable, shooting pain when breathing or moving the wrong way. I would describe the way I felt more in the category of discomfort.

"What restrictions will you have for the rest of your life?"
There are several foods I will never be able to eat. I am not allowed to garden due to bacteria in dirt. I am not allowed to change kitty litter or refill my bird feeders. Both activities can transmit bacteria.

Most of my restrictions have to do with infecting me. My immune system can't naturally fight off an infection because of my immunosuppression. If I get sick, I would have to take drugs: antibiotics, anti-virals, or anti-fungals. They boost my immune system so I can fight the infection. Unfortunately, my boosted immune system will want to fight off my heart, too. A bit of a conundrum, wouldn't you say?

As a final metaphor for how far someone can come, I thought it fitting to close out my book with some "before" and "after" photos. In years past, I would never have been comfortable sharing any of these. Given that the theme of this book is to be improve and inspire, I am happy to report that I have stepped outside of my comfort zone. If my vulnerability and publication of my journey of growth and acceptance can move you to get out of your comfort zone, this will have all been worth it!

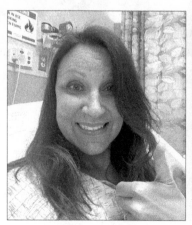 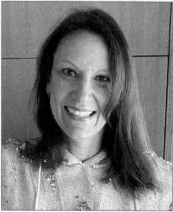

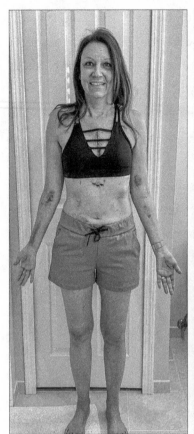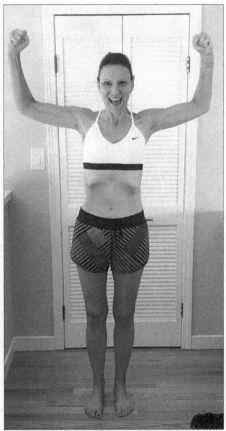

Epilogue

THE WELLNESS CHAPTERS AT the end of this book were meant as a high-level prompt for my readers. I wanted to encourage reflection, push some boundaries, provoke thought, maybe cause a little discomfort, and more than anything, encourage change. Each area of wellness I introduced has so much more dimensionality than I was able to capture in a few short chapters. I could write a whole other book to dive more deeply and really dissect human behavior.

Because I am not a psychologist, but because I feel so strongly that there are developmental opportunities for all of us, I have partnered with a psychotherapist on a future book. My ideas in this book were anecdotal, theoretical, and experiential. I hope you will join me in my next venture where "Dr. P." and I help you apply practices backed by years of research and clinical practice.

Watch this space!

Acknowledgments

THIS BOOK WOULD NOT be possible without the love, encouragement, and support of so many people. I need to express my deepest admiration for and thanks to...

My amazing husband, Dave Sidlar, not only for being my rock, but for allowing me to constantly fire questions at him when I was trying to recall details from my recovery. He is one patient human.

My mom, Marilynne Ponto, who has not only has been my #1 cheerleader during my entire heart health journey, but for being the most amazing caretaker after my transplant. And thank you to her significant other, Richard Paritzky, for letting me borrow her for 10 weeks.

My dad, Doug Balogh, stepmom, Linda Balogh, and brother, Marty Balogh, for constantly feeding me amazing book ideas, many of which have been incorporated into my writing and will be carried out as I continue to tell my story.

My medical team: Dr. Kim Man, Dr. David Lanfear, Nancy Amezcua RN, Dr. Hassan Nemeh, Dr. George Alangaden, Dr. Jennifer Cowger, and Dr. Alexander Michaels.

The staff at Troy Beaumont's Phase Two Cardiac Rehab, for the guidance and motivation, and for letting me loose for that first amazing run!

My post-rehab personal trainer, Nancy Kilkullen, for pushing me in all the right ways and building the confidence I was craving.

My incredible employer, The Mom Project, for providing an environment that allowed me to heal stress-free and return to my dream job.

Alicia Long and Kristi Piehl, for taking my story to the airwaves. I loved my podcast experiences with both of them.

My fellow Project Beautiful Inside and Out board member family, for continually lifting me up during my recovery and for creating a platform for me to introduce my Wellness Widget for the first time.

My Kappa Beta Phi sisters, who showered me with love and prayers and continue to be my constant support system.

My friend, Sam Ho, whose creativity and generosity were the inspiration for the title of my book.

The Detroit Writing Room and Stephanie Steinberg, for being an incredibly valuable resource during the unchartered waters of writing my first book. And thanks to Stephanie's mother-in-law, Sally, for planting the seed.

My graphic designer, Michelle Halliday, and my illustrator, Jodi Burton, for bringing my visual ideas to life. I love what they both created.

Sabrina Carrozza, my most generous public relations collaborator, and her team, Caroline Kasper and Michael LoRé. Sabrina's passion for women's heart health awareness and her drive to promote my book were inspiring and humbling.

Greg Sadler Photography, for the great 5K photos and his generosity in allowing me to use them in my book.

Talia Simpson and Kortney Pitts, for making my hospital homecoming so incredibly memorable.

Elizabeth Ann Atkins, writing coach extraordinaire, editor, publisher, podcast host, inspiration, and friend. Her hand-holding throughout my writing journey was more than I could have ever expected.

My dear friends and extended family, my lifeline, my tribe — for all the ways they lift me up, hold me accountable, push me, listen, and allow me to be me.

And the grandest of all thanks goes to my donor family. Their selfless gift, especially in a time of unthinkable grief, has meant more to me than I can ever express.

Kristy Sidlar Bio

KRISTY SIDLAR IS ON a mission to use her remarkable survival story as a heart transplant recipient to encourage men and women everywhere to make overall wellness a priority.

She's doing that through her memoir, *Change of Heart: My Journey of Transplantation, Revelation & Transformation*, by chronicling her victorious battle to survive as her heart failed.

Thanks to an organ donor family that was grieving the loss of their loved one, Kristy explores the power of gratitude and the inexpressible joy that the greatest gift of life can bring.

She also shares her Wellness Widget, a tool that she created to show how to improve your wellbeing by incorporating healthy habits into everyday life.

Kristy advocates for heart health, especially for women, as a long-time volunteer and board member for the American Heart Association. And she's a board member for Project Beautiful — Inside and Out.

Her career in the staffing and recruiting industry has enabled her to live and work in Singapore, and travel the world.

A Michigan native, Kristy has a Bachelor of Arts from Hope College. She and her husband, Dave, enjoy spending time in Northern California.

Kristy's hobbies include photography, fitness, card-making, and driving and admiring exotic and classic cars. After completing three 5K races since her surgery, she's currently training for a triathlon.

Please visit changeofheartmemoir.com.

Endnotes

1   Megan Call, "Why is Behavior Change So Hard?" U of U Health,
    February 14, 2020. https://accelerate.uofuhealth.utah.edu/resilience/
    why-is-behavior-change-so-hard

2   "Physical Wellness Toolkit," National Institutes of Health, last modi-
    fied August 26, 2021. https://www.nih.gov/health-information/physi-
    cal-wellness-toolkit

3   Richard O'Connor, Rewire: Change Your Brain to Break Bad Hab-
    its, Overcome Addictions, Conquer Self-Destructive Behavior, (New
    York: Plume, 2015). https://www.amazon.com/Rewire-Overcome-
    Addictions-Self-Destruc-Behavior/dp/0147516323/ref=sr_1_3?keyw
    ords=rewire+overcome+addictions+self+destructive+behavior&qid
    =1642124409&sr=8-3

CPSIA information can be obtained
at www.ICGtesting.com
Printed in the USA
BVHW061124310322
632995BV00003B/69

9 781956 879049